Two Knotty Boys

Back on the Ropes

D1476884

Two Knotty Boys

Back on the Ropes

A Step-by-Step, Illustrated Guide
for Tying Sensual and Decorative
Rope Bondage

JD and Dan, the Two Knotty Boys

Photographed by

Ken Marcus

Green Candy Press

Two Knotty Boys Back on the Ropes
by JD and Dan, the Two Knotty Boys
www.twoknottyboys.com
ISBN 978-1931160698
Published by Green Candy Press
www.greencandypress.com

Design: Ian Phillips
Cover image: Ken Marcus
Cover models: Heather Gates & Satine Phoenix

Printed in Canada by Transcontinental Printing Inc.
Massively distributed by P.G.W.

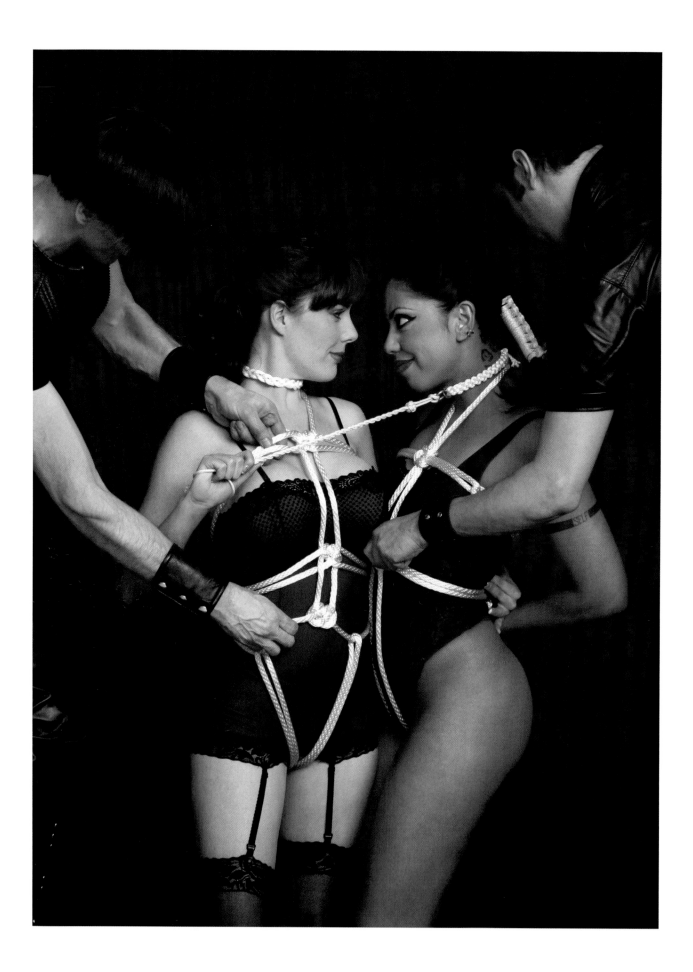

Contents

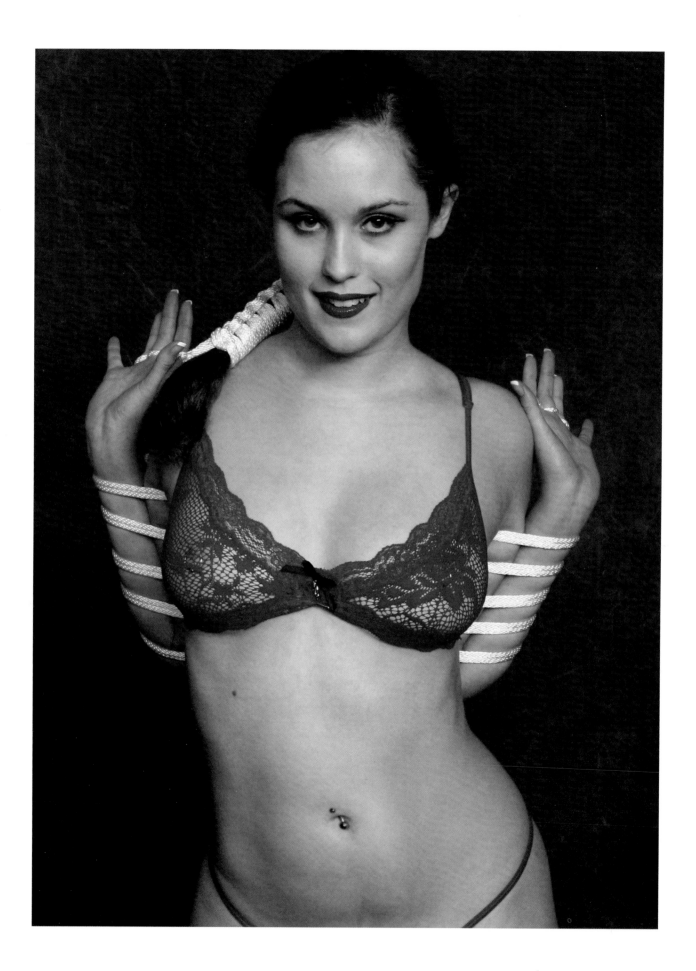

Foreword

Back in July of 2008 the Yerba Buena Center for the Arts, here in San Francisco, presented *CineKink*—a touring version of the erotic film festival that originated in NYC. On the second day of the festival *Coming Out Spanko* was featured. Created by, and staring, Tanya Bezreh, *Coming Out Spanko* is the video diary of a woman processing her sensual desire to be spanked (in a "deeply specific" way).

Throughout the fifteen minute long film, Tanya speaks directly to the camera, and so the viewer, expressing her fears, social hesitations and sensual needs with disarming honesty and emotional clarity. Watching this film, it's hard not to identity with Tanya and her quest for a more pronounced sensual identity.

Whether you're kinky, wiggly or straight, you have a heart—a heart that feels, wants and desires. So you can appreciate the magnitude of faith it takes to step out of the fold, hold your head up high and say, "I accept who I am, and what I desire." These are simple words; still they're words with profound meaning in a person's life. As Tanya put it, "To share it is to have faith. To share any true voice inside your body is to have a real faith."

There is a sensual desire within us all. In some cases a "deeply specific" one. Still most don't articulate their desires for fear of being judged, dismissed or forsaken. These fears are partially based upon feelings of isolation, or the belief that our immediate community (our town, city or region) does not possess like-minded individuals. But the horizons that formerly defined community have been broken. We are no longer bound by our towns, cities or regions. There is no longer a reason to feel alone or isolated. The Internet has united our world and the rope bondage community along with it.

You see, when we first started off on this crazy train called "Two Knotty Boys" we were teaching into a world of separated individuals—individuals whose communities were defined by their horizons. The year was 1999 and the Internet, although available, was still a relatively fledgling endeavor. Social networking sites, video sharing and podcasts were mere whispers of what they are today, and what they're fast becoming.

Generalist community networking sites have been co-opted and tailored to the specific interests of smaller, more topic centric groups. Video sharing has resulted in the creation of instructional videos, providing free access to information that was historically passed down person-to-person. Podcasts now provide weekly insights into the thoughts and ideas of people just like us.

Through our participation with social networking sites and the instructional videos we produce and post online, we've established connections with hundreds of thousands of individuals seeking to learn about and discuss the topic of sensual rope bondage. People from Iceland, Brazil, Germany, Denmark, Japan, Britain and Australia, as well as people from throughout the United States and multiple other countries of origin, no longer feel distant or far away. Technology has united us all in celebration of rope as a vehicle of connection.

Though the core of all life experience and exploration is personal, there exists a globally networked community of like-minded individuals that will support and embrace who you are—a community of one that plays as many. This truth has never been more evident than today, and it is our hope is for a more open, tolerant and compassionate world tomorrow. So as you turn through the pages of this book, exploring, learning, practicing and playing, remember this community; and, if you're moved to do so, share with them the personal joys and connections you experience through rope.

Thank you and keep tying,

—Two Knotty Boys

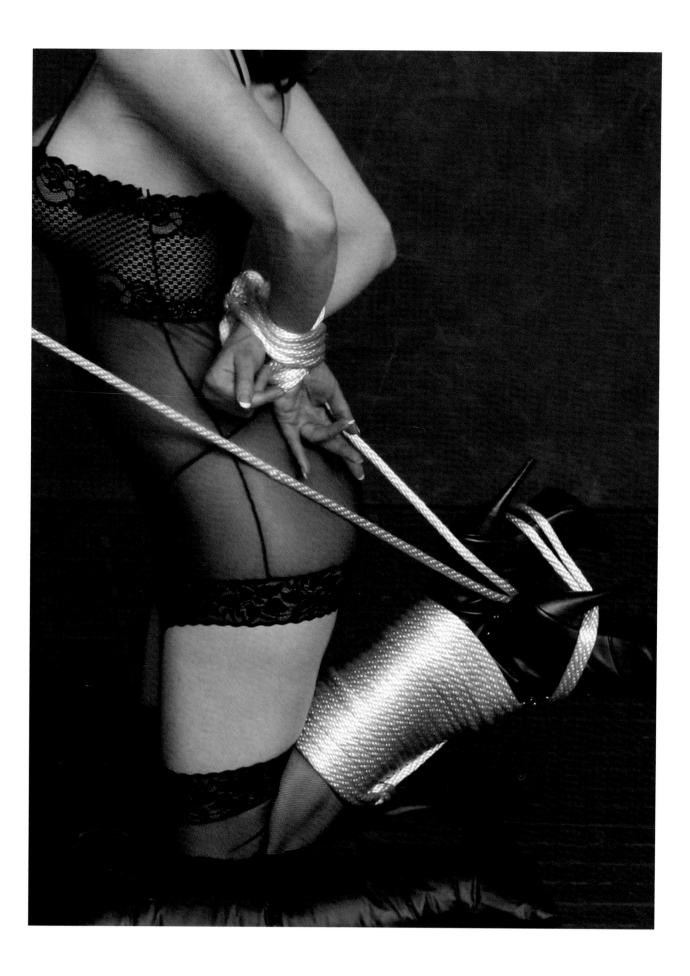

Acknowledgments

For cooperation with and/or inspiration in the production of this book, Two Knotty Boys would like to thank Ken Marcus, our models Heather Gates, Erin Sinclair, Satine Phoenix, Kapono Kobylanski, Miss Pixie, Twink, John Scott Trekauskas, Lexafina, Mina Meow, Charlotte Vale, and Stephan, as well as Simon Blaise, Lee Harrington, SubMissAnn, Cleo Dubois, Jahck, Steve Davis, David Goldburg, George Lazaneo (Bondage a Go Go), Eve Minax, Jimi Tatu, George Sandoval, Andrew McBeth (Green Candy Press), Peter Ackworth, Mistress Melissa, Mistress Snow, Master Feenix (and all the crew at Purgatory at Bar Sinister in Los Angeles), Jenni Romero, Sarah Ton and anyone who has ever hosted or attended a Two Knotty Boys workshop.

And...

A very special thanks to Kristen Kakos,
for your inspiration, patience, keen eye and sensibility.

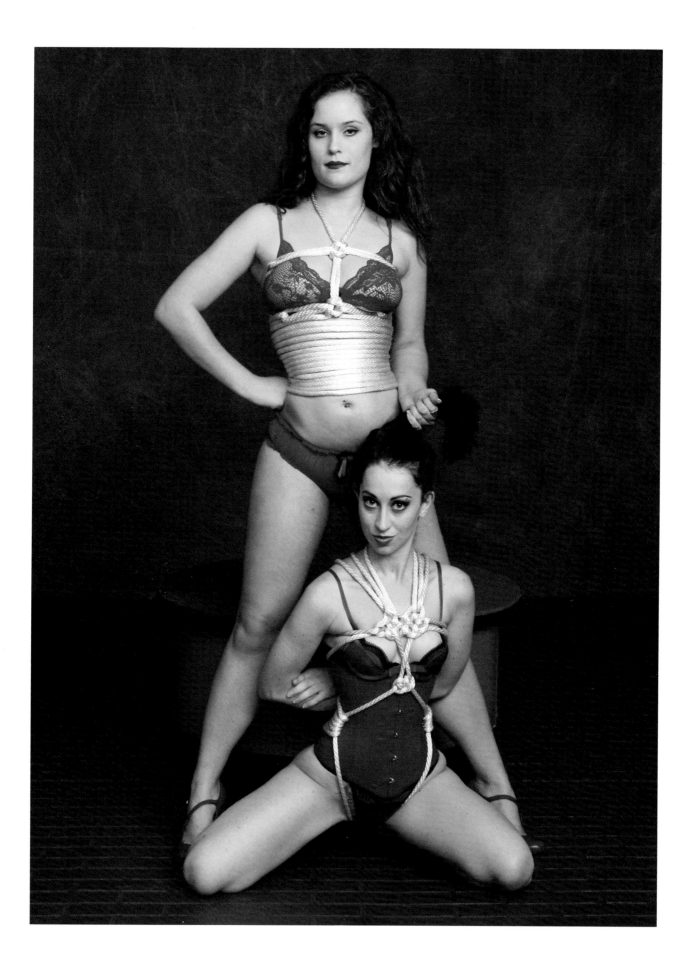

Introduction

Since teaming up as Two Knotty Boys in 1999, we've dedicated much of our lives to demystifying rope bondage. Our goal hasn't been to make bondage mainstream, but rather to put it within reach of anyone who has ever been inspired (or requested) to tie it and try it—whether for passion, fashion or BDSM play.

If you're interested in rope bondage, you're not alone. Researchers say that bondage is one of the most popular sensual fantasies. As *Psychology Today* notes, one in ten people has experimented with bondage. It is popular among men and women of all classes and educational backgrounds, according to psychologists and ethnographers.

Our first book, *Two Knotty Boys: Showing You the Ropes*, revolutionized rope bondage awareness and education by laying out the process using easy to follow, step-by-step photos and captions. Unlike videos or DVDs that you have to play, repeat and memorize, this format lets you learn at your own pace and refer to it as needed—even right in the bedroom or the dungeon.

Two Knotty Boys: Back on the Ropes does more than take up where *Showing You the Ropes* left off. It covers sixty-one ties—twenty-four more ties than we shared in our first book—and now it's in color. Best of all, we go beyond *Showing You the Ropes* by demonstrating how to use many of these ties and put them into action with your partner. In total, more than seventy rope bondage ties and techniques are revealed in the following pages.

When writing this book, we decided against making it an "Advanced Bondage" version or even "Volume II" of a set. While we're proud of the quality, content and contribution of *Showing You the Ropes*, we didn't want it to be a required purchase to enjoy this book. That's why we repeat the core knots, ties and techniques that we elaborate upon here in *Back on the Ropes*. Not only was this the easiest way for us to forge ahead and show you new applications, interactions and adaptations of these pieces, it was our way of assuring you purchased the first book because you wanted to, not because you had to. We have no interest in tying readers into a two-book deal—or forcing novices or intermediate players into a choice between one book over another.

We also insisted on pricing this book as reasonably as possible, regardless of the fact that it's in full color, with more models, features, ties and photographs than the first book. So much content and thorough coverage propels this book from the realm of guidebook into a veritable tome of ties.

With all that this book contains, you'll notice something it doesn't: fluff. For instance, we chose not to regale our readers with reams of rambling recitations about rope. Sure, you'll see a smattering of factoids about knot history and tradition, but we know that's not what you're here for. This is also not a book about dominance and submission. It is a tool kit. Whether you apply these techniques in a casual, playful or "drop to your knees and bow before me" kind of way, the choice is up to you. The same techniques will serve you equally well.

In a nutshell (or knot shell)…*Back on the Ropes* features beginning, intermediate and advanced knots, clever tricks, unique iterations of our foundation ties, decorative applications, ties for extra exposure, harnesses and more. The ties in this book will take advanced riggers to new heights and give novices more to look forward to. So whether you want to learn a few basic tricks just to try rope bondage on for size, or you want to wow your partner and anyone watching with your mastery of rigging, *Two Knotty Boys: Back on the Ropes* makes it more than possible. It makes it easy.

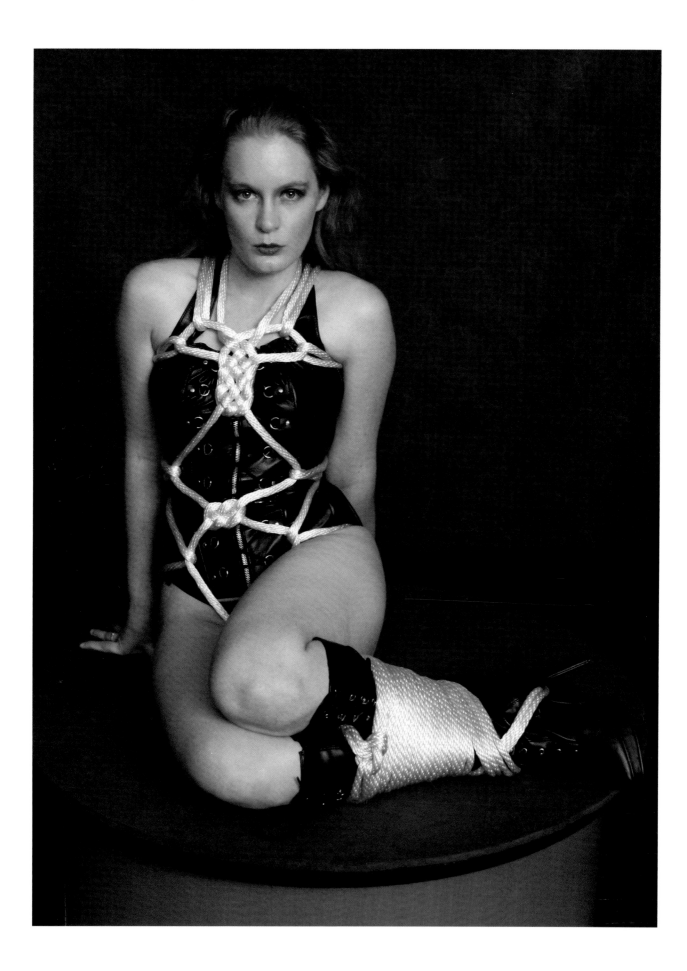

Rope Bondage Safety

The foundation of all safe and sensual bondage practices is compassion for the person you are tying. Compassion, or an awareness of and sympathy for the physical and psychological needs of your partner, will not only assure the sustainability of the connections you establish; it will assure you'll be playing for the rest of your life.

So please, before you even pick up rope, take the time to critically evaluate your feelings for the person you're about to tie. If you find yourself possessing the capacity to immediately and unquestionably respond to your partner's physical and psychological needs, proceed. If not, set your rope down and walk away.

Still reading? Good! It's time to learn about safety. The purpose of our books is to show you how to tie people—people with bodies, circulatory systems, nerves and sensibilities. On account of this fact, safe tying practices must be used during each tie outlined within this book, no exceptions.

Disruption of circulation is the primary safety concern related to rope bondage. This is because lack of circulation in any part of the body, regardless of whether it occurs in a region of a major artery or capillary network, can lead to tissue damage. Examples of tissue damage include bruising, temporary or permanent nerve damage and in extreme, unmitigated situations necrosis (tissue death).

Symptoms of a break in circulation include numbness, a tingling sensation, lack of sensation, a drop in skin temperature and a skin color change to pale white or blue. If the person being tied experiences pain or any of the symptoms listed above, remove the rope immediately!

Thankfully, none of the dangers associated with rope bondage are intrinsic; all are preventable with good techniques and sensible precautions.

The following are some common sense "Dos and Don'ts" that will help ensure safety during your rope bondage experience.

Rope Bondage DOs:

• **Do make restraints "two-fingers loose,"** or loose enough that you are able to work one or two fingers between the rope and the body.

• **Do monitor circulation every ten minutes.** Check for cooling of the skin or discoloration (usually whitening) on the limb beyond the binding. Let your partner know it's okay to tell you if anything starts to go numb.

• **Do insist your partner notify** you of symptoms of circulation loss immediately, such as numbness, tingling, "pins and needles" sensation or joint pain.

• **Do multiply the points of tension** to spread the effect over a wider area. Don't limit a tie-down to a bed, for instance, to attachments at the wrists and ankles; attach ties to the elbow, knees, shoulders, waist and thighs as well. The more widely you distribute the tension of a tie, the more exciting and safe that tie will be.

• **Do make sure you know how to undo** your ties before you put them on your partner. Be prepared to cut difficult knots or bonds in an emergency. To do this, keep safety scissors (also known as EMT shears or bandage scissors) handy at all times. They're available at most well-stocked drugstores.

• **Do go slowly** with novices and during first encounters. Be especially sensitive to your tyee's emotional reactions, providing frequent gentle body contact, spoken encouragement and reassurances. Watch out for developing panic.

• **Do remove restraints gently**, being careful not to cause rope burns. Lower the arms and legs so blood can flow in. Massage any area that has become numb; if necessary, apply warmth to restore circulation.

Rope Bondage DON'Ts:

• **Don't make any tie too tight**, especially around joints (wrists, elbows, knees, ankles) or the neck—anywhere that major arteries or veins are near the surface.

• **Don't leave someone** who's inescapably tied alone. Circulation problems can get very bad, very fast, not to mention what might happen if other medical emergencies occur or if the tyee struggles to a point of falling and injuring himself.

• **Don't gag your partner—unless** you provide an alternative method for them to communicate problems with circulation or other emergencies.

• **Don't attempt a rope suspension without proper training**, and never bind someone where support relies on a fixture, bolt or construction that has not been designed to bear a load many times that person's weight.

• **Don't let your ego get ahead of your better judgment.** Ego is the consciousness of your identity and is a necessary part of your self-awareness. However, if you connect your ego to your ties, requested adjustments or removals of the rope you've tied can lead to feelings of "wrongness," embarrassment or resentment toward your partner. These feelings can be reduced or avoided by remaining open to your partner's communicated needs and letting go of a "destination" or "goal" when it comes to play. The pursuit of an ideal or a "perfect" scene is the first step toward disconnecting with you partner. So let go, play safely and respond to your partner's needs with compassion, always.

• **Don't let your partner's submissiveness interfere with safety.** Even though you have stated your need to be informed of circulation loss or "bad" (distracting or unintended) pain, be aware that your partner may try to "tough it out" to impress you, fall into an uncommunicative, hypnotically submissive state of mind (known as "sub space") or succumb to "get-tied-itis" disease, a condition in which people are so eager for bondage that they ignore safety.

For these reasons, it's essential that you keep checking in with your partner throughout the experience, especially if you notice unusual or reflexively defensive physical responses to the ropes, such as increasingly frequent or intense twisting of the wrists or ankles.

The Knots

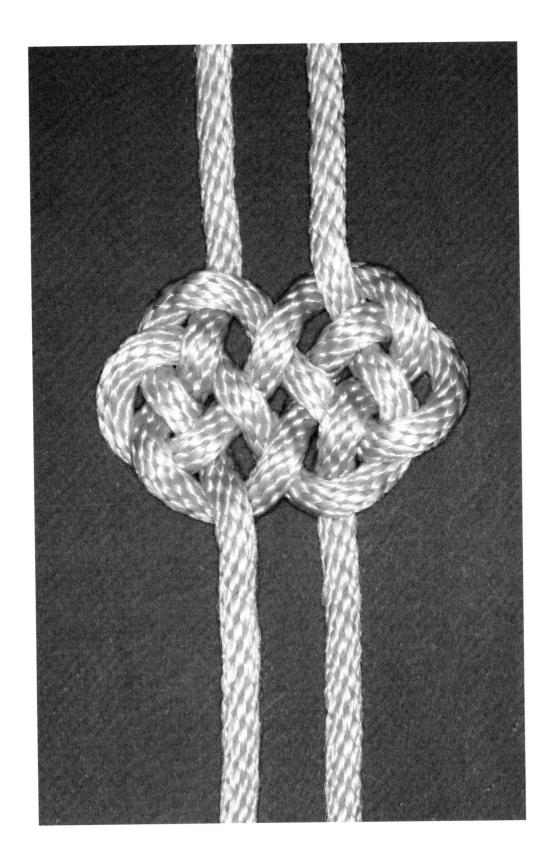

Square Knot

This is the knot behind the rhyme "right over left, left over right makes a knot both tidy and tight," still it can be tied with either rope end leading first. The most basic of the flat knots, it's quick and easy to tie, and a secure way of finishing off a piece. If you're a martial artist, you may recognize this knot as the one used to tie the Obi (or belt). A drawback to the knot is its ability to come undone when one of its working ends is pulled outward. So maintaining even tension on the working ends is vital to the knot's usefulness.

Rope length: Any length
Rope diameter: Any diameter

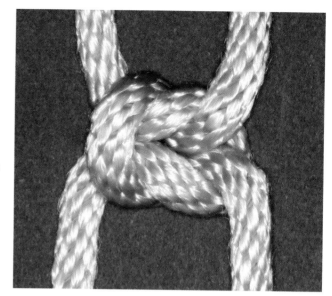

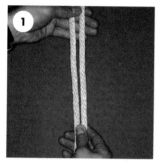

Start with two rope ends dangling side by side.

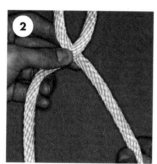

Cross the RIGHT rope over the left rope.

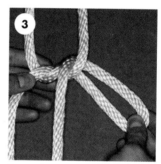

Bring the rope on the right-hand side up and tuck it over the front of the loop created.

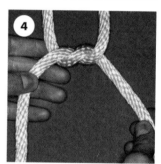

Notice, once again you have two rope ends dangling side by side.

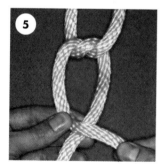

Now cross the LEFT rope over the right rope.

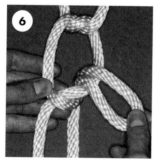

Bring the rope on the right-hand side up and tuck it over the back of the loop you just created.

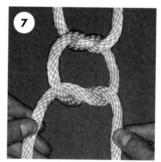

Tighten the knot by pulling the rope ends firmly.

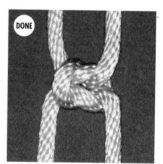

You'll know you tied the knot correctly if the top of the knot and the bottom of the knot are parallel to one another.

Split Square Knot

Essentially a Square Knot tied around two standing ends of rope, this knot will prove its worth when finishing off our body harnesses. The fundamentals of a Square Knot are two half knots (also called overhand knots), alternating right and left or left first and then right. The Spilt Square Knot maintains the functionality of this knotting technique while incorporating the structural integrity of two taut ropes.

Rope length: Any length

Rope diameter: Any diameter

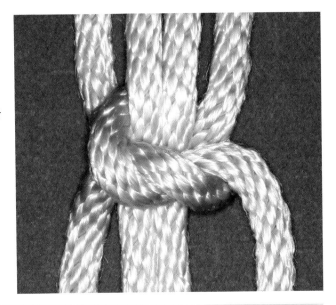

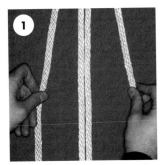

Start off with two rope ends dangling side by side alongside two taut ropes (shown in the middle).

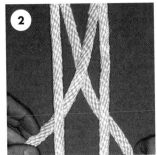

Behind the taut ropes, cross the right rope over the left rope.

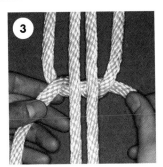

Bring the rope on the right-hand side up and tuck it over the front of the loop created.

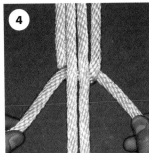

Pull the rope ends downward firmly.

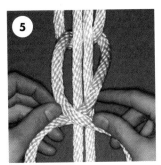

In front of the taut ropes, cross the left rope over the right rope.

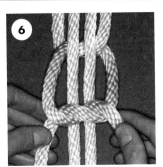

Bring the rope on the right-hand side up and tuck it over the back of the loop created.

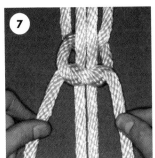

Tighten the knot by pulling both rope ends firmly.

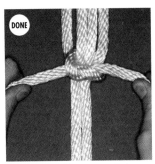

The top and bottom of the finished knot will be parallel to each another, but the knot itself will sit horizontally.

Double Slipknot

Slipknots are also called "running" knots because the knots "run" (or slip) along the rope and can be easily untied by pulling the working ends. The Double Slipknot comes in handy when tying the wrists or ankles of a person who has limited flexibility. The knot needs to be properly hitched off to stop its tendency to tighten as strain is put upon it.

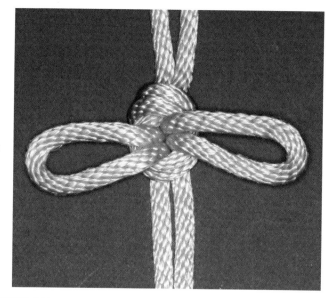

Rope length: Any length
Rope diameter: Any diameter

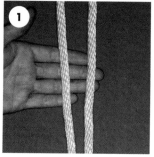

1 Start with two rope ends dangling side by side.

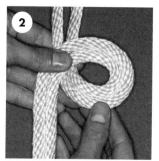

2 Gather the ropes into a pair and rotate them up and over themselves into a counterclockwise circle. Make sure the "leg" of the loop is in front of the *P* shape you created.

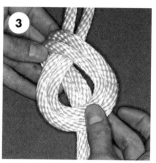

3 While holding the looped rope firmly in one hand, slide the dangling pair of ropes behind the loop.

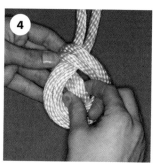

4 Reach through the front of the loop and pinch the pair of ropes behind it.

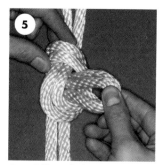

5 Carefully pull the pinched ropes through the loop.

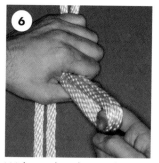

6 With one hand, grip the knot at the base of the protruding double loops. Then hook the double loops with the finger of your other hand and pull them toward you.

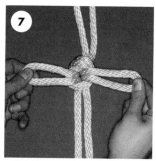

7 Split these protruding loops apart, and...

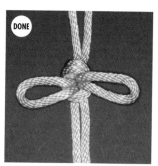

DONE there you have it: a Double Slipknot!

True Lover's Knot

This knot takes its name from the legend that Dutch sailors tied it to remind themselves of their loved ones during long ocean voyages. The knot is the product of two intertwining overhand knots (symbolizing two intertwined lovers) and is the centerpiece of our Lover's Harness. Remaining firm when pulled tightly, the knot can be incorporated into a variety of ties and maintains its decorative appearance under struggle.

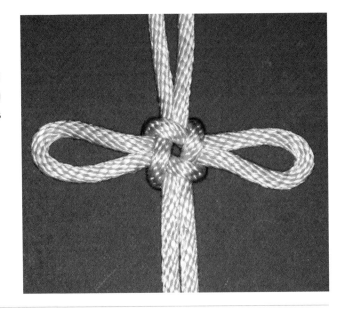

Rope length: Any length
Rope diameter: Any diameter

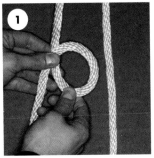

1 Start by making a counter-clockwise loop. Make sure the "leg" of the loop is in front of the P shape created.

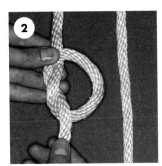

2 Tuck the "leg" behind and through the loop it made.

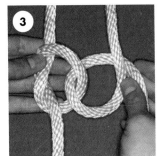

3 Take the other dangling rope and rotate it clockwise. Pass the end of this rope through the front of the loop on the left side and back behind itself to make a q shape.

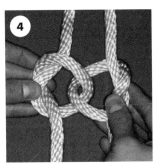

4 Now tuck the "leg" of the q down through the front of its own loop. You now have two overhand knots linked together.

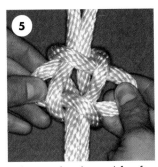

5 Fish your thumbs and forefingers between the left and right overhand knots and pinch the opposing center loops.

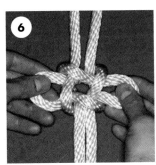

6 Gently pull the opposing loops until they emerge out the sides.

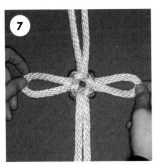

7 Pull the loops firmly, cinching them in place.

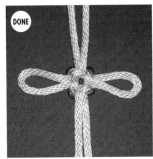

DONE Now you're ready to tie a lover!

Double Coin Knot

This is our signature knot! We use it in more ties and in more ways than any other knot in this book. An Asian knot, it mimics the appearance of two antique Chinese coins overlapping. Merchants once believed the design of the knot brought prosperity and a prolonged life. Extremely versatile, the knot is the foundation of other knots and can be tied using doubled lines for a larger, more elaborate appearance. In all truth, a book could be written on just this knot and its myriad applications.

Rope length: Any length
Rope diameter: Any diameter

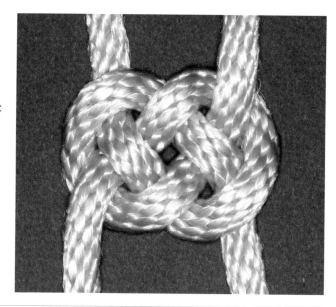

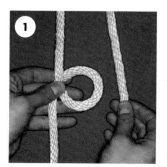

1 Start by making a counter-clockwise loop with the left rope. Make sure the "leg" of the loop is behind the *P* shape you created.

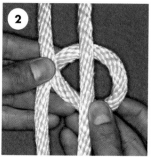

2 Keeping the loop open, place the right rope over the *P* so it looks like a pencil in front of an eye.

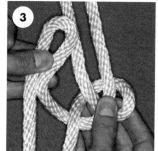

3 Transfer everything into your right hand. Pinch the *P* together to maintain its shape. Create a bight in the right rope and pass it under (behind) the "leg" of the *P*.

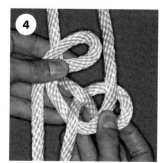

4 Weave the bight over (in front of) the upper left rope. Make sure the right hand still holds the "pencil" rope in front of the "eye" loop.

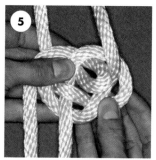

5 Tuck the bight under the top of the *P* and out through the front.

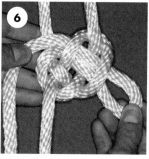

6 Now dive the rope over the "pencil" and down through the open loop on the lower right corner. Finish the knot by pulling the bight's rope entirely through the knot.

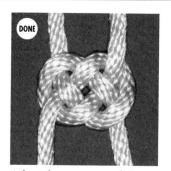

DONE Adjust the ropes carefully throughout the knot to make sure it's flat and looks symmetrical. Don't try to tighten the knot by pulling on both ropes or it will collapse.

Box Knot

Elements of this knot lend themselves to a variety of beautiful flat knots, the Long Knot and the Temple Knot, to name a few. Still, it is also quite useful in its own right. Fiendishly effective at gripping fingers and toes, it is our favorite knot for connecting rope to an extremity. Beyond this, its most useful quality, it also makes a beautiful addition to a chest harness or decorative wrap.

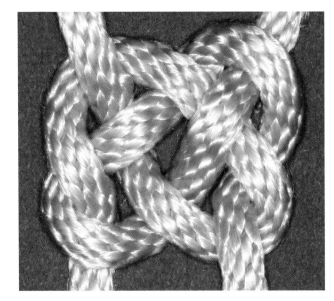

Rope length: Any length
Rope diameter: Any diameter

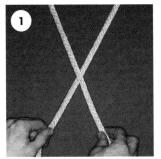

1 Cross the left rope over the right rope.

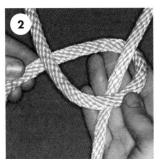

2 Rotate the rope on the right-hand side up and behind the ropes above in a counterclockwise loop. Make sure the "leg" of the loop is BEHIND the *P* shape you created.

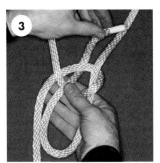

3 Turn your attention to the dangling rope. Rotate it clockwise and insert it through the loop of the *P* above.

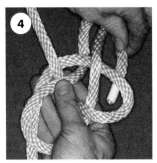

4 Now weave the rope over the rope to its right, then behind and through the loop immediately below it.

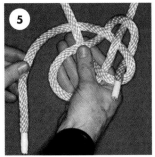

5 Turn your attention to the left-hand rope and…

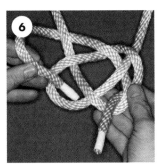

6 tuck it through the front of the loop below it.

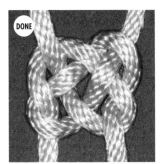

DONE Well done. You have just completed the Box Knot!

Long Knot

This knot takes the base of the Box Knot and runs "long" with it. Essentially this knot is a weaving technique that could extend to any length desired. However, for the purpose of creating our Butterfly Harness, it is best tied as illustrated below. Still, there's no need to limit the use of this knot to harnesses. You can use it for a variety of other pieces too, including bracelets and collars.

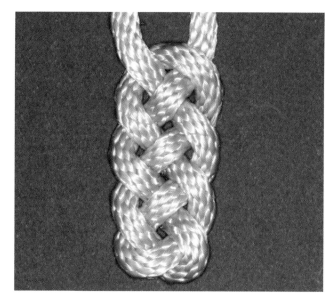

Rope length: Any length
Rope diameter: Any diameter

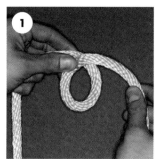

Start by making a downward loop. Make sure the right-hand rope lies on top of the loop you created.

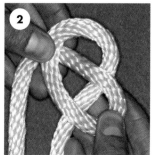

Fold the right rope down, behind and across the back of the loop.

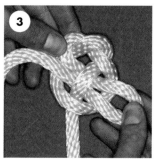

Form a bight in the left-hand rope and weave it over the left side of the loop, under (behind) the middle rope and over the right side of the loop.

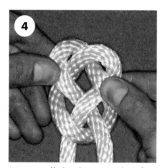

Now pull the loose side of the bight until the end of the rope pulls all the way through the knot.

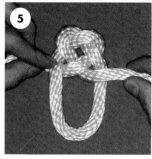

Widen the loop until it hangs down about 3 inches (8cm) long.

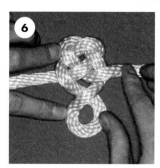

Twist the loop so that the right side crosses down over the left.

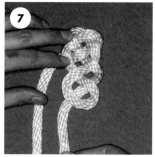

Fold the right rope down, behind and across the back of the loop.

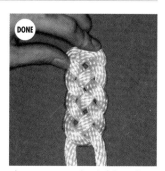

Then, weave the left-hand rope over the left side of the loop, under the middle rope and over the right side of the loop.

Temple Knot

This knot's name is derived from its similarity to the appearance of a Buddhist temple crowned by a stupa (or spiritual monument). A simple extension of the Box Knot, when tied it takes on a unique appearance that we feel surpasses the beauty of its derivation. Still, like the Box Knot, it makes a visually impressive addition to a chest harness or many other creative applications.

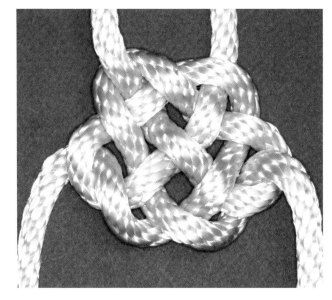

Rope length: Any length

Rope diameter: Any diameter

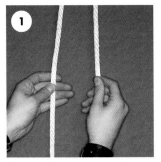

Start with two rope ends dangling side by side.

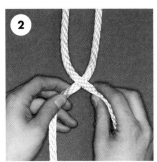

Cross the left rope over the right rope.

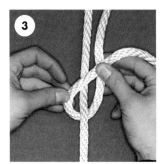

Fold the left-hand rope up, over and across the top of the loop created.

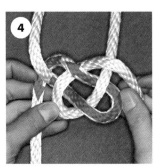

Weave the right-hand rope under the right side of the loop, over the middle rope, and under the left side of the loop.

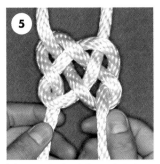

Now tuck the left and right working ends over and through, then under and through, the left and right bottom loops. At this point, you've created a Box Knot.

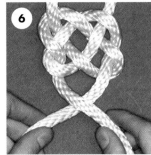

Once again, cross the left rope over the right rope.

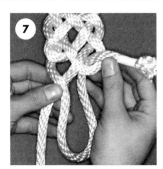

Tuck the right-hand rope under and through the lowest loop of the Box Knot.

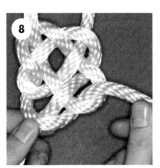

Make sure to pass your working end between the diagonal rope and the outer right edge of the Box Knot's lowest loop.

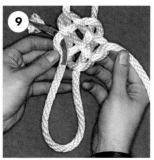

9

Repeat Steps 7 and 8 using the left-hand rope, but this time, tuck the rope over and through the lowest loop.

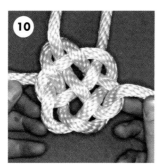

10

Adjust the knot...

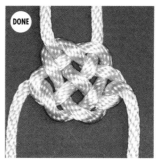

DONE

until it takes on the sacred appearance of the Temple Knot.

Rabbit Knot

This knot takes its name from the fact it looks like a rabbit when completed. Effectively, it is a Box Knot tied with two equal-sized bights. Aside from its fluffy connotation, the knot is a useful addition to a chest harness or any other tie that you might wish to improve by incorporating an ornate, detached knot. If you think of the Rabbit Knot as a technique, it can be applied to a variety of knots to incorporate bights in place of the working ends of a rope.

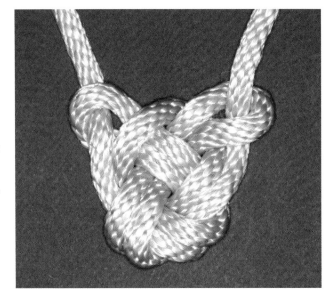

Rope length: Any length

Rope diameter: Any diameter

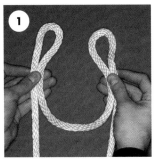

Start off by dropping the rope into an *M*, creating two equal-sized bights on either side.

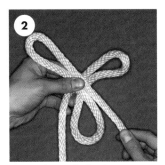

Cross the right bight over the left bight, making a loop at the bottom.

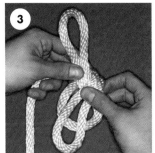

Fold the right bight down, over and across the top of the loop below it.

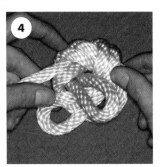

Now fold the left bight down, behind and over the bight that bisects the loop under it.

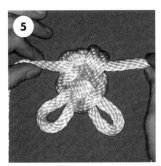

Then, tuck the left bight down through the right edge of the loop.

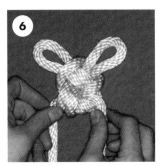

Flip the knot upside-down.

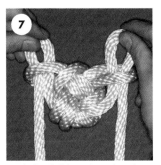

Tuck the left-hand and right-hand ropes up through the front and back of the left and right bights, respectively.

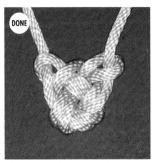

There you have it...the Rabbit Knot!

Flower Knot

The name of this knot reflects its simplistic beauty and floral appearance. A sequential variation from a number of different knot families, it is referred to as "Hana Musubi" (or Flower Knot) in Japan. Useful when seeking to create a harness that sprouts off of a knot maintaining two or more available loops, it makes an elegant centerpiece.

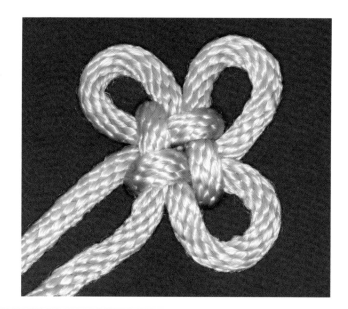

Rope length: Any length

Rope diameter: Any diameter

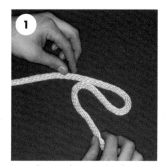

1 Start by making a bight, or a single loop, pointing toward the right.

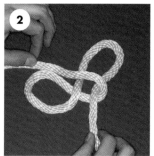

2 Below this bight, make a second bight and insert it up through the first bight you created.

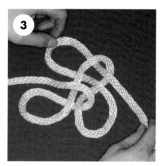

3 Create a third bight and tuck it up through the second bight you created.

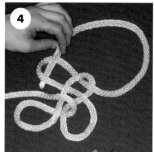

4 Now take the working end of the third bight and weave it down through the bight it created...

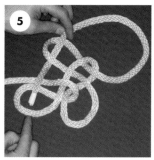

5 then over both lines of the first bight...

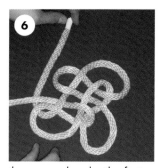

6 then up and under the first bight.

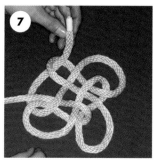

7 Finally, tuck the working end of rope up underneath and through the third bight.

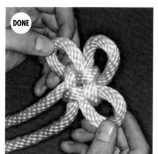

DONE Adjust the piece by pulling on the "petals" of the knot while taking up any slack within the knot.

Prosperity Knot

This knot is based on the Double Coin Knot. More specifically, it is an extension of a Double Coin Knot, creating the appearance of multiple "coins" stacked upon each other. Such is the reason why the knot was given the connotation of prosperity or wealth in China. For our purposes in this book, the Prosperity Knot is the centerpiece of the Prosperity Glove, Belt Buckle and the Chest Plate Harness.

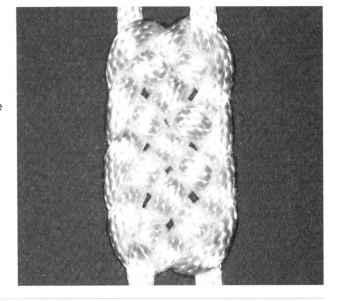

Rope length: Any length

Rope diameter: Any diameter

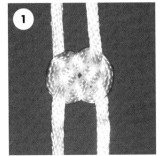

Start by tying a Double Coin Knot.

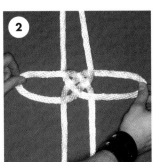

Stretch the left and right loops of the Double Coin Knot out 4 inches (10cm) to create the appearance of "wings."

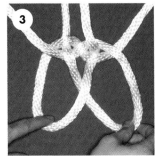

Move the left and right working ends of the rope upward above the loops.

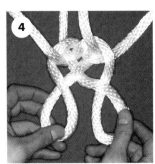

Twist both loops clockwise (left over right).

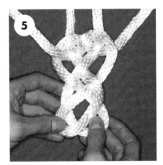

Cross the right-hand loop over the left-hand loop.

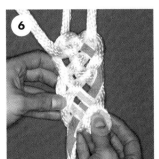

Then, bring the right-hand rope down from above and weave it first over the right-hand loop and then underneath the left-hand loop.

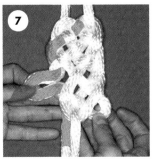

Now make a bight in the left-hand rope and weave it underneath the outside left bulge of the left-hand loop...

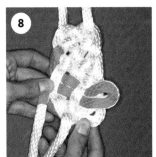

and over the left side of the right-hand loop, then under the right-hand rope...

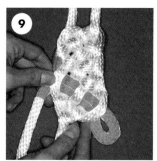 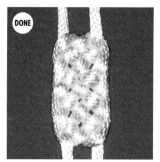

over the right side of the right-hand loop, and finally, under the outside right bulge of the left-hand loop.

Take a breath, adjust your knot, and congratulate yourself. You just finished the second most difficult knot in the book!

Challenge Knot

You guessed it; this knot is a "challenge." Still, its beauty and Celtic elegance make it a noble addition to a rigger's arsenal of flat knots. Whereas most of the knots previously described lend themselves to one another, this knot stands alone. Don't be intimidated by this knot's uniqueness or its name for that matter. It's very doable and you will impress your partner and wow people once you tie it in front of them—or better yet, show them how it's done.

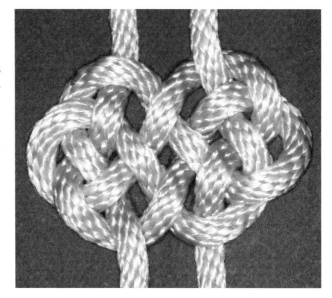

Rope length: Any length
Rope diameter: Any diameter

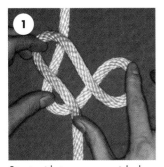

1 Start with two ropes side by side. Shape the left-side rope as shown by first making a backward J, making a bight in the lower rope and laying the bight up across the J.

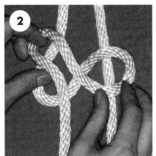

2 Drop the right-side rope down and under the twisted loop that protrudes to right side of the left-hand rope.

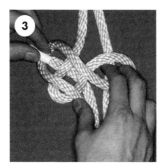

3 Begin weaving with the end of the right-hand rope. First weave underneath the lower left bight and out through the loop created by the upper left bight.

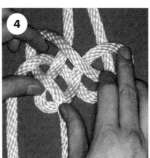

4 Now weave the working end down and...

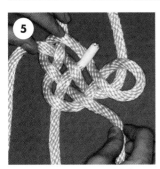

5 underneath the lower left bight, over the rope crossing the lower left bight and under itself.

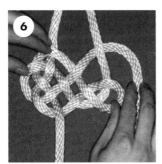

6 Continue by weaving the working end over the upper left bight again, and under the upper right standing end of rope.

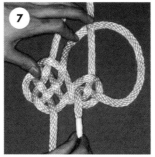

7 Drop the working end down and over the right loop, under itself over the right loop again...

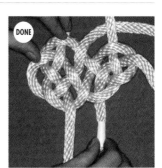

DONE and under itself a final time. Now congratulate yourself. You have met the challenge successfully!

Sliding Sheet Bend

Also called the Mooring Hitch, the Sliding Sheet Bend is a quick and easy way to secure a partner's wrists or ankles to a fixture or an eyebolt. Strong and dependable, the knot can slide (hence the name) allowing you to increase or decreases the distance between a tie point and the limb of your partner. When the fun is done, all you have to do to undo the knot is pull a "ripcord," exploding the hitch instantly!

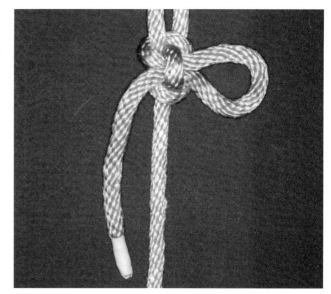

Rope length: Any length
Rope diameter: Any diameter

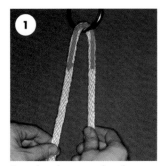

1 Start by drawing the short end of the rope (sliding it from right to left) around a fixture or through an eyebolt.

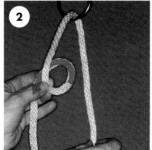

2 When the short end of the rope is two feet (60cm) down from the fixture, make a P-shaped loop in the short rope, turning it counterclockwise and under itself.

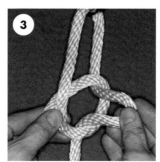

3 While holding the P in place between your thumb and forefinger, lay the loop over the long rope. Then reach through and pull a short bight through the loop.

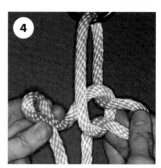

4 With your left hand, make a bight in the short rope under the P. Insert this bight through the bight in the long rope you previously pulled though the loop.

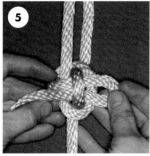

5 Pull the left bight one or two inches (3 – 5cm) through the right bight.

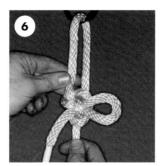

6 Flatten the knot and cinch it tighter by pulling down on the long end of the rope, so the bight in the middle "chokes" the bight that goes through it.

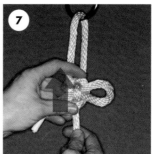

7 To increase the slack or length of the standing end (in this case, the long part of the rope), pull down on the standing end with one hand, while you slide the knot up.

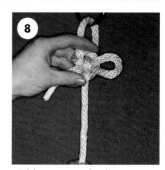

8 Holding on to the knot overcomes the friction that prevents the knot from sliding when the standing end is pulled.

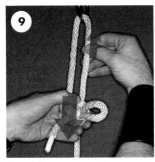

9 To add tension or shorten the standing end of the rope, hold on to the standing end (above the knot) and pull it up while you slide the knot down.

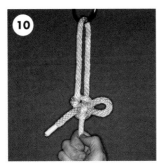

10 When you let go of the knot, the hitch remains secure even when the standing end is under tension.

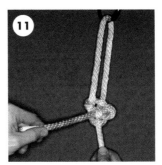

11 When you're ready to undo the tie, simply pull on the short rope (or "ripcord") dangling from the knot.

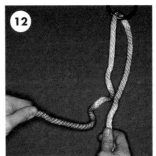

12 Watch as the knot disappears instantly, like magic...kinky, kinky magic.

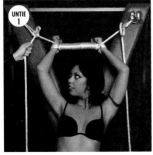

UNTIE 1 Seen here in its natural environment, the Sliding Sheet Bend, in conjunction with the Basic Wrap, provides a nifty way to tie someone to a Saint Andrew's cross.

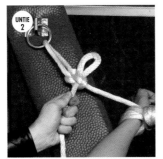

UNTIE 2 When your partner has done enough time on the cross...

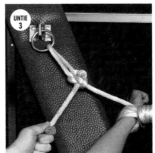

UNTIE 3 simply pull on the "ripcord" and the knot comes undone.

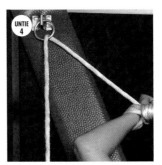

UNTIE 4 Your partner comes down with both wrists still bound for more fun to come!

Clever Tricks

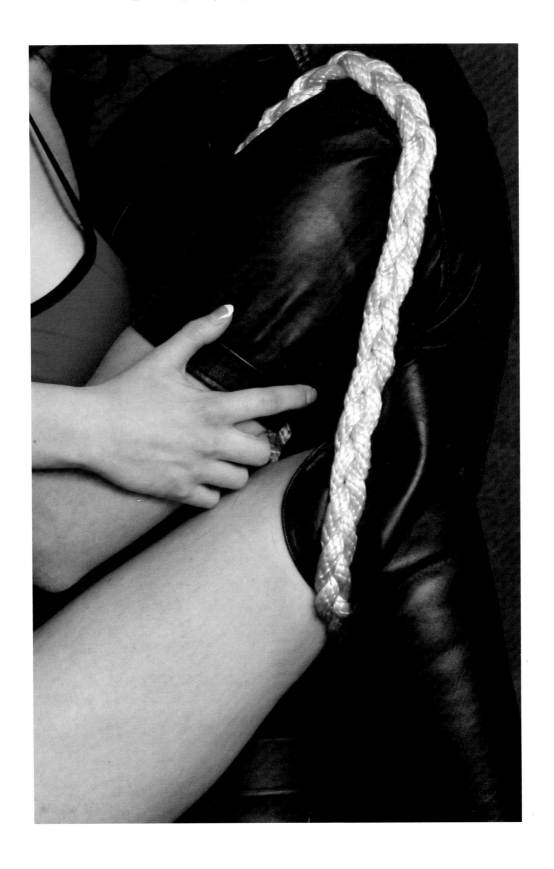

Rope Strap

The Rope Strap is the modification of a braid called the Australian Plait. Its subtleness belying its versatility, it can be used to thicken a section of thin diameter rope while avoiding the potential for pinching and constriction. The technique also has other uses that we show later in Rope Strap Applications.

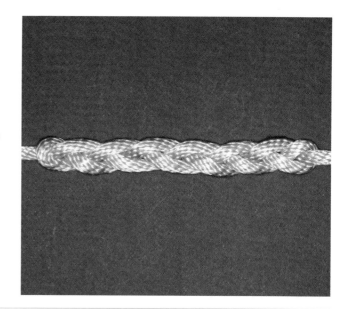

Rope length: 10 to 20 feet (3 – 6m)
Rope diameter: ⅜ to ⁷⁄₁₆ inch (9 – 11mm)

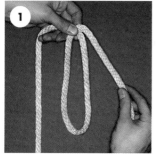

Start by making a dropped loop. Make sure the right-hand rope end is on top of the loop created.

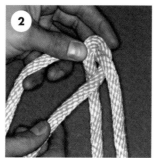

Tuck the right working end of rope behind and through the dropped loop.

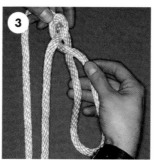

Twist the loop clockwise, left over right.

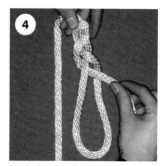

Tuck the working end behind and through the dropped loop.

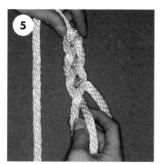

Twist the loop counterclockwise, right over left. Then tuck the working end behind and through the dropped loop.

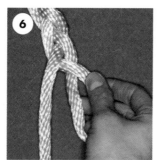

Twist the loop clockwise, left over right. Then tuck the working end behind and through the dropped loop again.

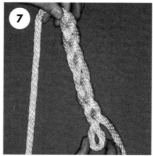

Continue this alternating technique all the way down the dropped loop...

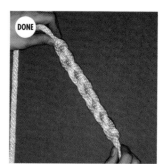

until you reach its end. Once there, your strap is complete!

Rope Strap Applications

Applications of the Rope Strap abound, and in all truth, you only have to dig into your imagination to discover multiple uses for its simple yet elegant design. Still, to kick-start your adventures, we decided to present a handful of ideas that we hope will get your creative juices flowing!

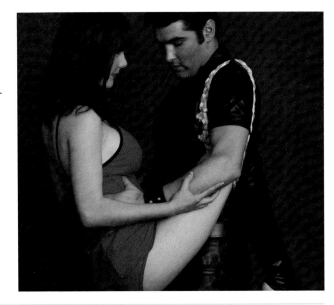

Rope length: 10 to 20 feet (3 – 6m)
Rope diameter: Various

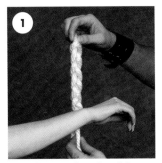

Ready-Made Shackle
(⅜ inch or 9mm rope)
Start by tying a Rope Strap long enough to wrap around your partner's wrist or ankle.

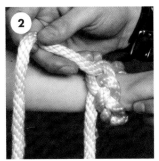

Tuck one of the working ends through the last loop on the opposing end of the Rope Strap.

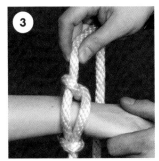

Tuck the other working end through the last loop on the end of the Rope Strap opposing it.

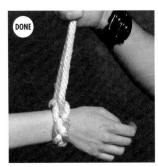

Done! The wrist is up to you.

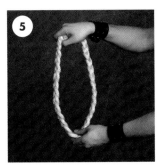

Standing Sex Strap
(⅜ inch or 9mm rope)
Make a Rope Strap long enough to loop from your shoulder to your hip. Tie the ends together with a Square Knot.

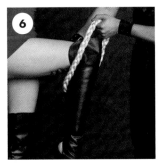

Have your partner step into the looped strap, drawing it up to the thigh.

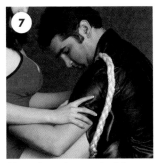

Sling the other end of the strap over your corresponding shoulder...

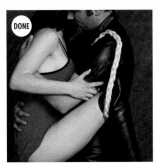

and step in close for hands-free action!

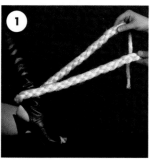

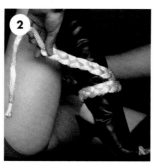

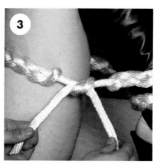

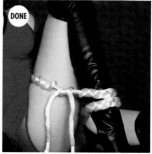

Quick Thigh Strap
(³⁄₈ inch or 9mm rope)
Tie a strap long enough to wrap 1½ times around your partner's thigh. Place the strap around the back of your partner's ankle.

Cross the strap ends in front of your partner's shin, wrapping one end of the strap around the inner thigh and the other around the outer thigh.

Tie off the strap with a Square Knot.

Now your partner can't kick or extend the leg.

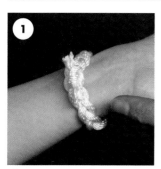

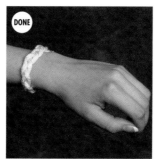

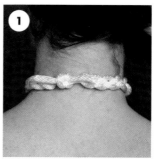

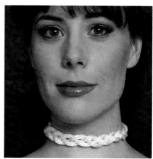

Elegant Bracelet
(⅛ inch or 3mm rope)
Start by tying a Rope Strap long enough to circle your partner's wrist. Tie off the piece with a Square Knot...

and cut off the excess rope for braided bracelet.

Elegant Collar
(⅛ inch or 3mm rope)
The same technique as the bracelet can be used around the neck using a longer length strap...

to create an elegant collar or choker.

Switchback Rope Strap

Many riggers choose to use thin diameter rope when performing hikes, partial and full suspensions. Under such circumstances, experience leads most to increase the number of coils around a limb to better distribute the body weight supported. However, even in the hands of the most experienced rigger, coiled rope occasionally pinches and constricts, causing discomfort and ultimately a loss of circulation. The following technique is intended to address this concern, increasing the surface area of a rope, while reducing the potential for pinching and constriction.

Rope length: 10 to 20 feet (3 – 6m)
Rope diameter: $^3/_{16}$ to $^1/_4$ inch (3 – 6mm)

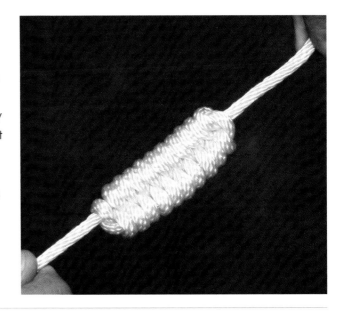

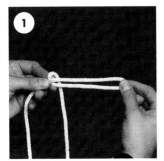

1 Start by making a dropped loop. Make sure the right-hand rope end is beneath the loop you created.

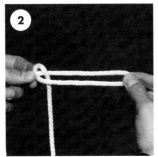

2 Tuck the right-hand working end of rope over and through the dropped loop.

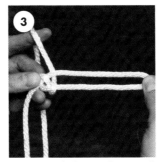

3 Again, tuck the working end over and through the dropped loop.

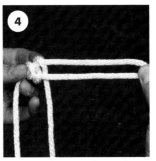

4 Keep performing Steps 2 and 3…

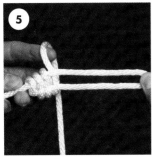

5 down the loop…

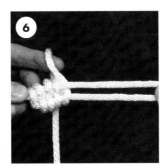

6 until you reach…

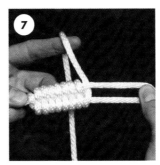

7 the loop's end.

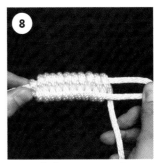

8 To cinch the piece in place, hold on to the standing end of the rope…

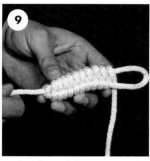

and pull it while you grip the rope strap.

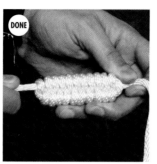

If your rope strap looks like the tail of a rattle snake, all is well.

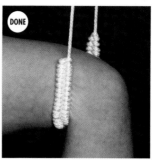

Here's how it looks supporting the thigh.

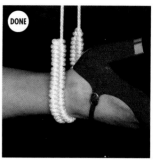

Here's how it looks supporting the ankle.

French Bowline Shackle

In contrast to our Rope Shackle, a tie that requires two working ends to complete, the French Bowline Shackle only requires one working end of rope. At first glance, this may not seem significant, but as you start to play with combinations of our ties, the usefulness of this shackle will become more apparent.

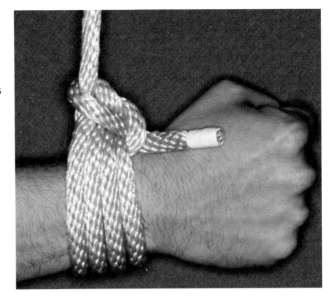

Rope length: 10 to 15 feet (3 – 5m)
Rope diameter: ³⁄₈ to ⁷⁄₁₆ inch (9 – 11mm)

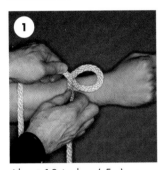

About 18 inches (.5m) up from the end of the rope, make a counterclockwise loop on the limb of your partner. Make sure the "leg" of the loop is in front of the P shape.

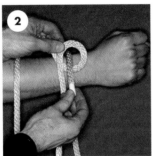

Wrap the leg of the P around the limb and through the loop.

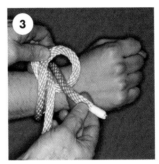

Repeat Step 2...

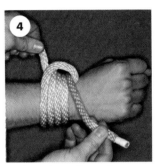

until you've achieved your desired number of loops around the limb.

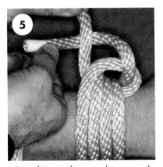

Now bring the working end of rope up and around the back side of the long standing end of the rope.

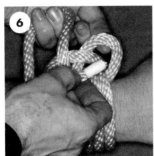

Tuck the working end back through the loop of the P and parallel to itself.

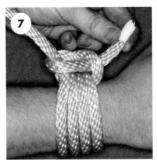

Pulling on the working end while holding the standing end...

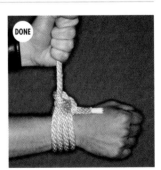

cinches the piece in place. Like the song says, "Love shackle, baby, love shackle!"

Cross-Armed Bow Knot

If you've tied your shoes, you've tied a bow knot, a quick and easy technique for "handcuffing" a person's wrists together. Still, we're about to show you a clever new way to tie this knot that you likely haven't imagined. Taught to us by a sailor we met in a London pub called The King's Head, this slick cross-armed technique will be sure to impress bar buddies and partners alike!

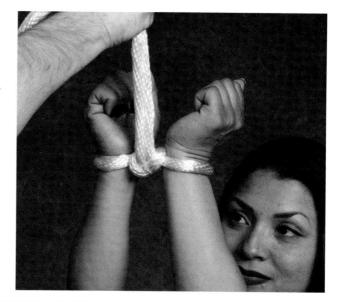

Rope length: 10 feet (3m)
Rope diameter: ¼ to 7/16 inch (6 – 11mm)

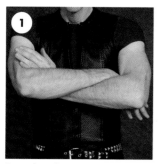

First, lay the rope over your partner's parallel out-stretched arms. Now, cross your arms so that one hand is above and one hand is below.

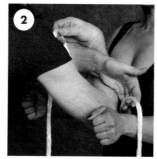

Approach the rope on your partner's arms. With your arms still crossed, pick up one rope with your right hand and the other with your left hand.

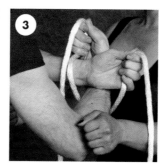

While holding on to the ropes, carefully uncross your arms. Don't let go of the ropes!

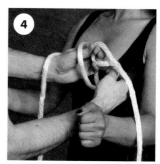

Carefully pull your hands apart, allowing the ropes to slide across your wrists and over your hands.

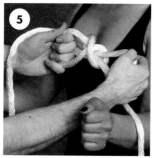

As you pull your hands farther apart, you'll notice a knot forming between two gripped loops (or bows).

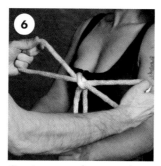

Continue stretching out the loops of the bow until the knot is tight.

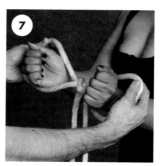

Immediately pull the completed loops back towards you and then slip them over your partner's still-outstretched wrists. Because the bow knot is a Double Slip Knot...

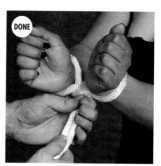

you can cinch the loops around your partner's wrists by holding the knot in place and pulling on both working ends. Now your partner is ready for you to take the lead!

Prisoner Cuffs

The one thing we hear most about the following piece is how quick and easy it is to complete. Still, don't let that fact lull you into complacency. There are subtleties associated with this tie, subtleties that if not fully understood will lead to frustration. That said, the Prisoner Cuffs rock! Quick to tie when mastered, the cuffs are an awesome way to add a sprinkle of fantasy to role playing or dynamic exchange.

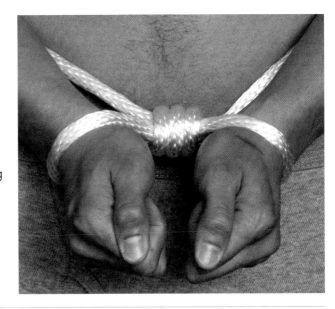

Rope length: 10 to 15 feet (3 – 5m)
Rope diameter: ³/₈ to ⁷/₁₆ inch (9 – 11mm)

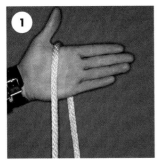

Start winding your rope around your hand about six inches (15cm) before the middle of your rope.

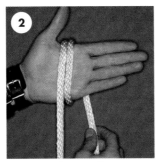

Keep winding until...

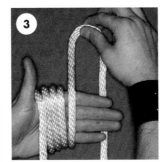

you've completed four winds around your hand.

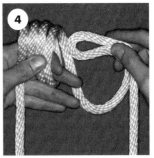

While pinching the winds side-by-side, make a bight in the right working end of the rope and carefully tuck it...

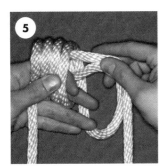

into and...

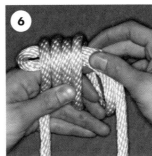

through all the loops you created.

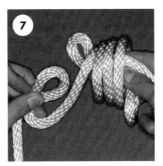

Repeat Steps 4 through 6 using a bight created in the left working end.

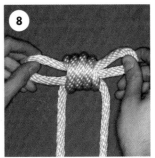

At this point you should have a tie that looks like two "rabbit ears" poking out of the sides of a barrel.

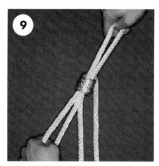

Pull the "rabbit ears" apart firmly.

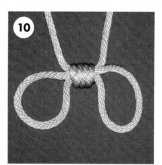

This locks the winds tight around the looped ends.

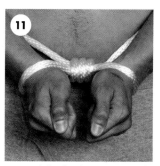

Now slide the loops around your partner's wrists, pulling on the left and right working ends to secure the piece. Keep a two-finger space between the loops and the skin.

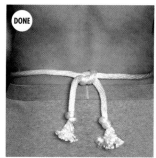

Finish off the piece using a Square Knot tied in the back.

Quick Gripper

A novel application of the Prisoner Cuffs, the Quick Gripper is one of the fastest and most effective ways to bind your partner's arms, upper arms or ankles. The functionality of the piece is complemented by how easily it is fixed in place and how difficult it is to remove by the person cinched within its grip!

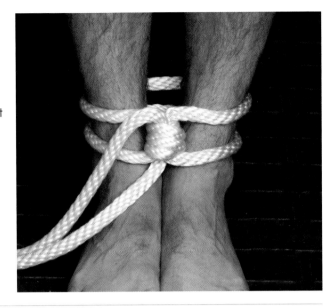

Rope length: 10 to 15 feet (3 – 5m)
Rope diameter: ³/₈ to ⁷/₁₆ inch (9 – 11mm)

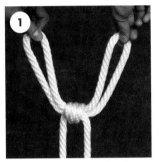

Begin by tying a pair of Prisoner Cuffs, making sure both loops of the cuffs are equal in size.

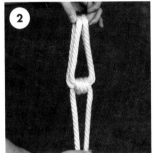

Bring the loops of the cuffs up so that they're in line with the working ends of the piece.

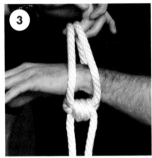

To bind the wrists, slide both loops of the piece over one wrist, then...

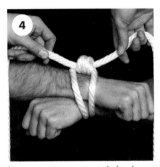

have your partner slide the other wrist into the loops in the opposing direction. Pulling on the working ends locks the piece in place.

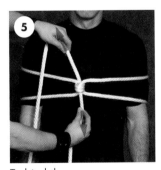

To bind the upper arms against the body, slide the loops of the piece over the shoulders and down across the chest. Split the upper and lower loops across the arms.

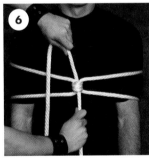

With the working ends lined up in the middle of the chest, pull! The arms cinch against the torso.

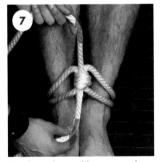

Binding the ankles is similar to binding the upper arms, only you're sliding the upper and lower loops over the feet.

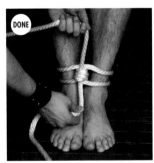

Pulling the working ends locks the piece in place! As with all of our ties, make sure to maintain enough space for two fingers between the ropes and your partner's skin.

Zip Snare

A common challenge to quick, effective restraint is the fact that most knots slip when struggled against. Such knots rely on loops that cinch tighter as they're pulled upon, restricting circulation and leading to discomfort. However, sliding knots are the most convenient for securing rope around a limb. So how can you keep a sliding knot from moving once you've placed it where you want it? How do you also create an adjustable loop that doesn't collapse around a limb? The answer is the Zip Snare! It's ideal for bedpost bondage and other times you're out on a limb for quick, safe, easily removable and struggle-proof bondage.

Rope length: 10 to 15 feet (3 – 5m)
Rope diameter: ³⁄₈ to ⁷⁄₁₆ inch (9 – 11mm)

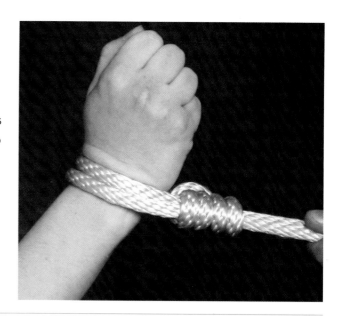

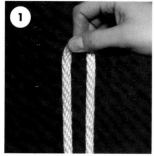

Start with a bight at the middle of your rope.

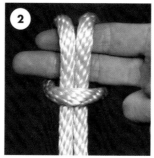

Then pass both ropes around your fingers and through the bight.

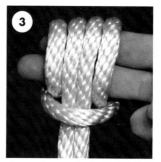

Wrap the working ends of the rope around and though the bight a second time, this time passing between the previous ropes on each side.

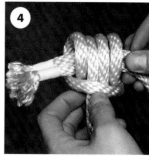

Now take the working ends of the rope and tuck them through the opening in the wraps previously around your finger.

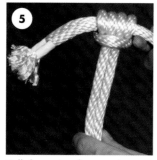

Pull the pair of ropes that drop beneath the bight, cinching the wrapped ropes firmly around the working ends.

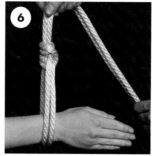

Slide the cinched wraps of rope down until you've made a medium-sized loop.

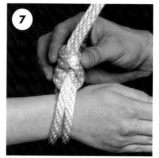

Slide the cinched wraps up or down to whatever position you desire, to loosen or tighten the loop.

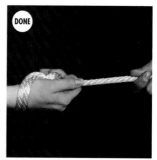

No matter how hard your partner pulls, the loops shouldn't loosen, collapse or tighten! However, you can free your partner at any time by sliding the wraps to open the loop.

Monkey Fist Ball Gag

Just in case you didn't already know, we love gags! We love how they fill our partners' mouths, muffling their voices, rendering them silenced and feeling vulnerable. We love all these things and we love rope. So we thought hard and long about a gag that would make for a formidable stifling of sound, even in the largest of mouths. What we came up with was the Monkey Fist Ball Gag. It's big. It's eye catching. It's also better tasting than an actual monkey's fist (so we hear).

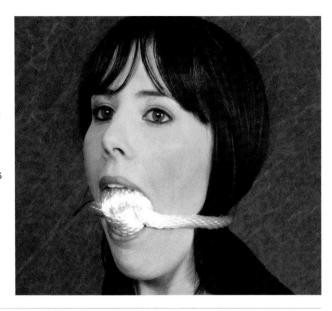

Rope length: 10 to 15 feet (3 – 5m)
Rope diameter: ³/₈ to ⁷/₁₆ inch (9 – 11mm)

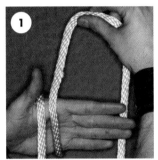

Start winding your rope around your hand about 12 inches (30cm) before the middle of your rope.

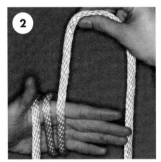

Keep winding until...

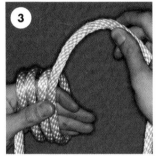

you've completed three winds around your hand. Pinch the winds so that they remain parallel to one another.

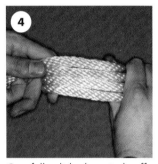

Carefully slide the winds off your hand and rotate them 90 degrees.

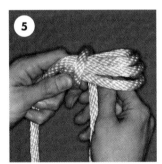

Now begin winding the right working end of rope up and over the horizontal winds of rope.

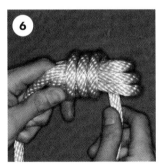

Once again, keep winding until you've completed three winds.

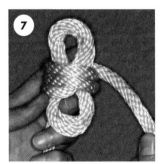

Rotate your winds 90 degrees until you see what looks like an *8* with horizontal wraps around its middle.

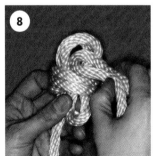

Tuck the working end through the top loop of the *8*.

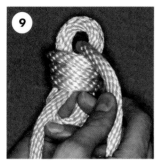

Pull the rope straight out through the other side.

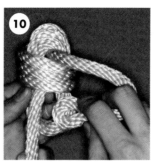

Then tuck it down through the lower loop of the *8*.

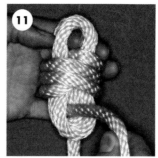

Once again, pull the rope out through the other side.

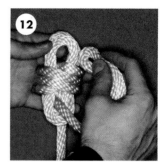

Repeat Steps 8 through 11...

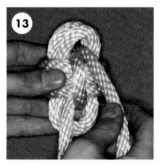

one more time.

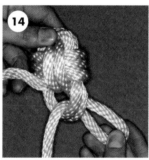

Finish two winds before...

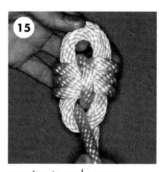

pausing to make your...

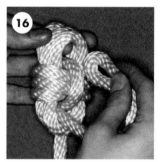

final adjustments.

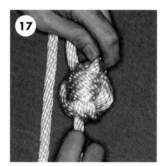

The final adjustments include working out the slack and...

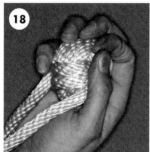

shaping the ball...

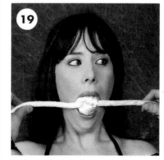

before fitting the gag in place, and...

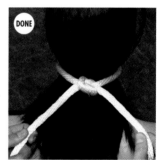

tying the piece off with a Square Knot.

Thick Bit Gag

In our first book, *Two Knotty Boys: Showing You the Ropes*, we showed you how to tie the Quick Bit Gag. Through continued play and comments from fans of the piece, we discovered that it works best when tied on people with small mouths. Not all people have small mouths, and not all people with big mouths can handle the size of a Monkey Fist Ball Gag. In response to this reality, we came up with the Thick Bit Gag, a smart and effective compromise between our large and small rope gags...and one that any smart mouth will find effectively compromising.

Rope length: 5 to 10 feet (1.5 – 3m)
Rope diameter: ³⁄₈ to ⁷⁄₁₆ inch (9 – 11mm)

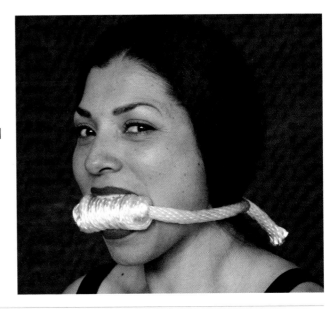

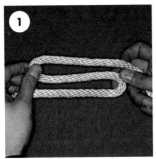

1. Make an *S* shape with your left and right working ends. Make sure the width of the *S* is equal to the length of your partner's jaw.

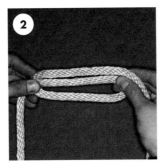

2. Rotate the bottom bend of the *S* up, so that the left working end creates a loop.

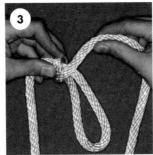

3. Now start coiling the right working end over the loop beneath it.

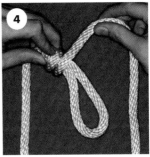

4. Make sure each coil made is parallel to, and tightly pressed against, the coil next to it.

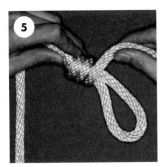

5. Keep wrapping until...

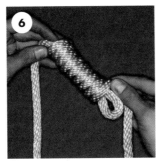

6. you reach the end of your loop.

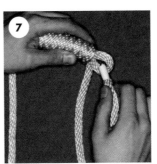

7. To lock the piece in place,

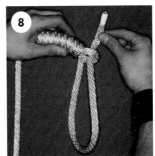

8. tuck the working end into...

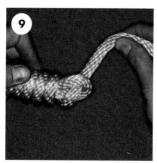

and through the loop end.

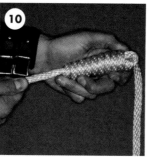

Pulling on the opposite working end...

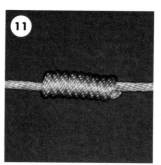

cinches the piece in place.

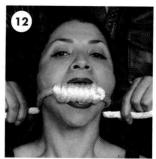

Tying the piece off is easy. Just wrap the ends of the gag around your partner's head and...

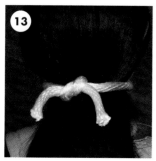

tie them together with a Square Knot.

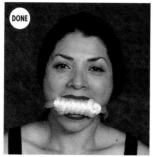

We've heard of sight gags, but this gag is a sight to behold!

Unique Iterations

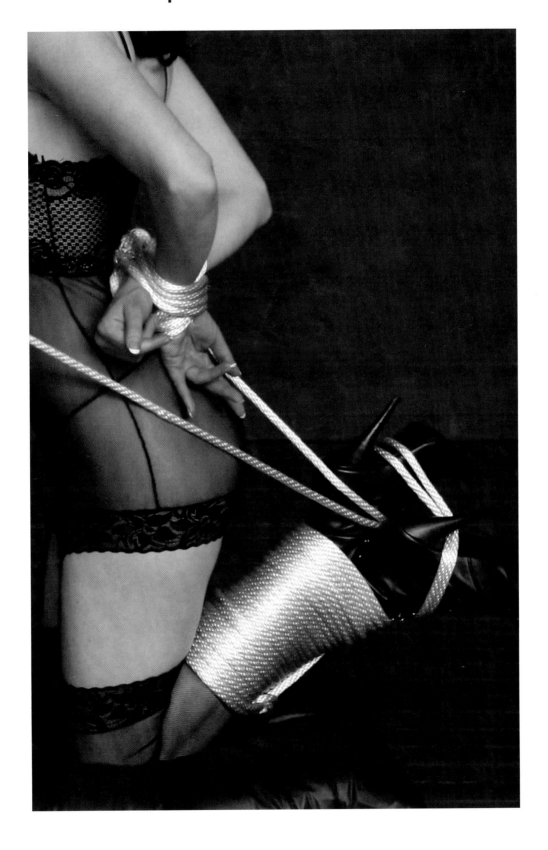

Cat's-Paw Stirrup

The Cat's-Paw is a wonderful way to secure a foot onto a bed. Still, the tie is also great for lifting a foot up to toward an eyebolt, canopy bed, shower rod or chandelier. It takes mere seconds to tie and it is comfortable enough to spend hours playing doctor, boot worshippers, puppeteer or crane operator. Oh come on…surely you've played crane operator? There's simply no simpler way to get a leg up on your partner!

Rope length: 15 feet (5m)
Rope diameter: 3/8 to 7/16 inch (9 – 11mm)

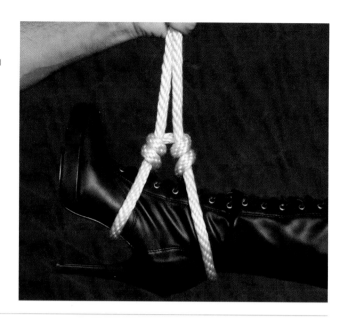

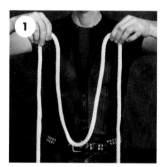

1 With both hands holding the rope a little wider than shoulder-width apart, droop the middle of the rope to make an M for "Meow, I'm a Cat's-Paw."

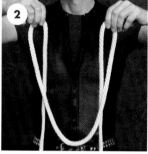

2 Using the tips of your fingers, twist the loops in opposite directions.

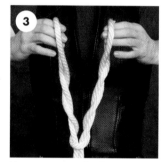

3 Keep twisting the loops an equal number of times.

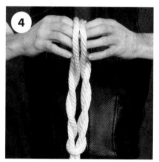

4 Then, bring the twisted loops together side by side.

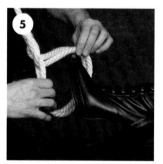

5 Hold the loops open wide enough to fit over your partner's boot or foot. Now ponder for a moment, why doesn't "boot" rhyme with "foot?"

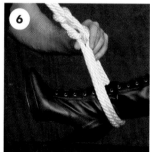

6 Slip the Cat's-Paw over the ankle.

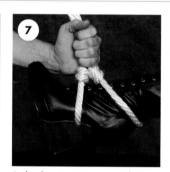

7 Split the Cat's-Paw so that one loop rests under the arch of the foot and the other rests behind the ankle. Secure the piece by sliding the twists down to the foot.

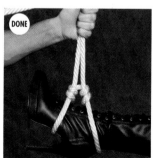

DONE Attach the working ends to a fixture or eyebolt overhead to lift and support the foot.

Cat's-Paw on Bare Foot

It's a well known fact that the Cat's-Paw for ankles works best when it's tied on a person wearing boots—long, formfitting thigh-high boots! Okay, we should come clean. Aside from our love of rope, we also have a (not very secret) love of boots. Nevertheless, we understand that tying a booted ankle isn't for everyone. Some people prefer bare feet, yet still wish to spread their partner's legs effectively, inhibiting the ability to close the knees or "pigeon toe" to block advances. We're putting our foot down that bare feet are sexy too!

Rope length: 5 to 10 feet (1.5 – 3m)
Rope diameter: 3/8 to 7/16 inch (9 – 11mm)

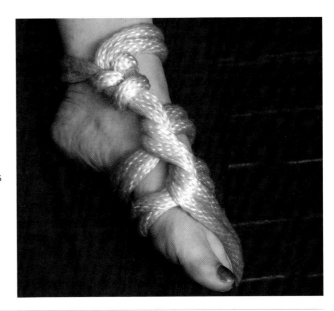

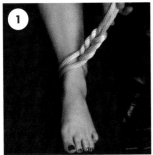

Begin by tying a Cat's-Paw large enough to easily slip around your partner's ankle.

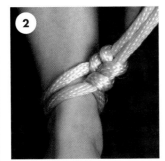

Slide the Cat's-Paw's rope bundles down toward the ankle until you achieve the look of a rattlesnake's tail.

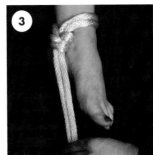

Now bring the working ends of rope toward the inside arch of your partner's foot.

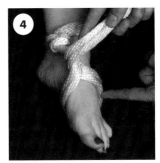

Wrap the working ends under the arch, around the foot and under the ropes stretched along the instep.

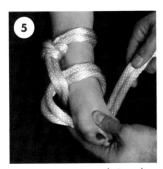

Repeat Steps 3 and 4, only this time wrap the working ends under the front pad of your partner's foot.

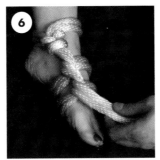

Bight the working ends back toward the outside edge of the table or bed your partner is lying on.

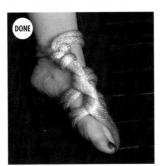

With what remains of your working ends, fix your partner's foot in place by tying off the working ends to a post or slat.

Rope Flogging Cuffs

When setting up another for a flogging, the most typical tie-off is at the wrist, at best with rope directed across the palm for extra grip and support. However, under the intensity of play, bottoms tend to relax into their bindings, resulting in an unsafe amount of weight bearing down on their wrists. In consideration of this reality, we created the following. It's a simple yet effective tie that supports weight while distributing it evenly through the whole hand.

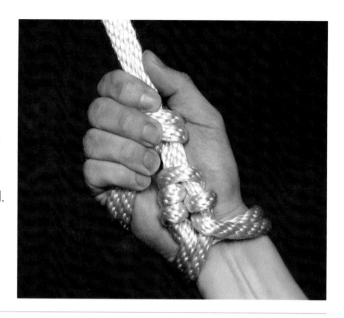

Rope length: 5 to 10 feet (1.5 – 3m)
Rope diameter: ³⁄₈ to ⁷⁄₁₆ inch (9 – 11mm)

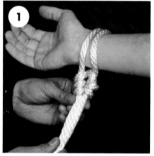

Start by tying a Cat's-Paw and placing it around the wrist of the person being tied.

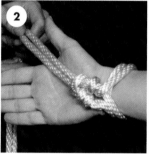

With the Cat's-Paw branching off the inside of the wrist, stretch the running ends diagonally across the palm between the forefinger and thumb.

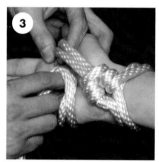

Now wrap the running ends around the back of the hand and across the palm.

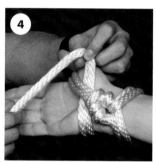

Tuck the running ends under the ropes stretched diagonally.

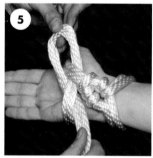

Then tuck the running ends over and under themselves...

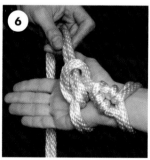

and through the loop you created.

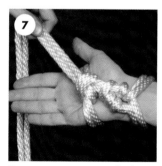

Remove any excess slack before cinching the palm knot firmly.

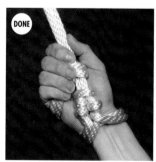

Once tied off, the piece safely and effectively supports the wrist. However, never attempt to use these cuffs to uncomfortably stretch or lift a person off the ground.

Rope Shackle *(Tied in Hand)*

The Rope Shackle is a terrific way to tie an arm or a leg to a fixture, a piece of furniture or even another part of the body. It's also useful for adding support to a suspension. The multiple loops of the shackle spread force equally, making it more secure and more comfortable. The elegance of the piece is that it doesn't tighten up under weight or when struggled against. As we described in *Showing You the Ropes*, the shackle can be tied directly onto a person. Now we're going to show you how to tie it ahead of time, in your hand, so you can more skillfully slip it over the body part you want to secure.

Rope length: 12 feet (4m)
Rope diameter: ¼ to ⁷⁄₁₆ inch (6 – 11mm)

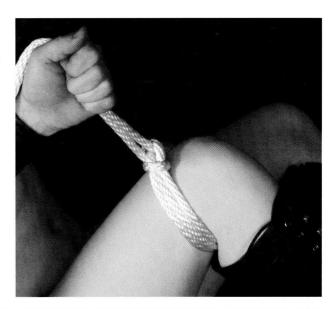

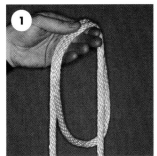

Start by making three or four equal-sized loops...

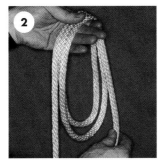

large enough to go over the body part you're planning to secure.

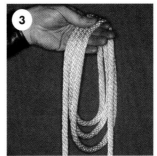

If you're using thinner rope, use four or more loops to more effectively support the weight resting on the rope.

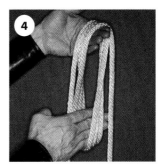

One you've decided on the proper number of loops, tug on the bottom of them all to assure they're equal in size.

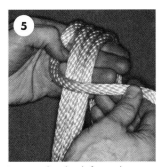

Now take the left working end of the rope and bend it around your thumb to make an *L* so that the rope passes over all the loops.

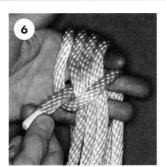

Bring the working end of the rope underneath all the loops (except for the left-most loop) and pull it out through the inside corner of the *L*.

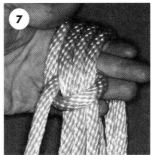

Tug the rope all the way through and let it hang down toward you.

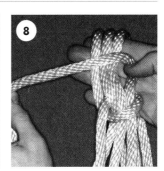

Now take the right working end of the rope and make a *7* with your thumb in the corner and crossing over all the loops.

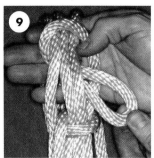

Pull this working end of the rope under all the loops except for itself, pulling it out through the opening in the 7 beneath your thumb.

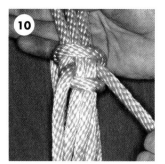

Now you have symmetrical hitches across all the loops.

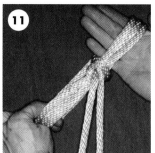

You'll adjust the size of the finished shackle once it's placed over the body part you're going to tie.

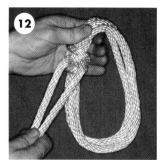

The pre-tied shackle stays intact, so you can tie several of them ahead of time and store them in your rope bag for quick use later as needed.

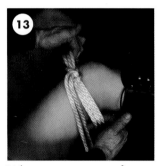

When your partner is fit to be tied, slip your pre-made shackle over the body part you want to secure.

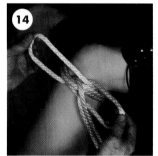

Once in place, adjust the size of the loops by first pulling outward on the hitches that cross over the loops. As you pull, the loops slip and begin to tighten around the limb.

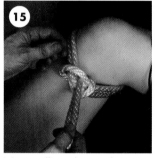

Now pull on the working ends of the ropes to take up the slack and collapse the hitches back onto the loops, re-forming the knot.

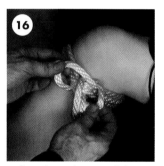

Refine the tightness of the shackle by successively pulling on the hitches (or "ears" of the knot)...

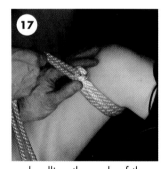

and pulling the ends of the rope as you hold on to the knot and pinch it together. Be sure to allow enough room for a finger or two to slip between the shackle and the skin...

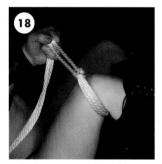

to help maintain blood circulation. Pull gently on the shackle to avoid any sudden jerks that could injure nerves. (Otherwise, you might be the jerk your partner avoids.)

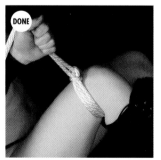

You'll find this to be one of the most versatile and useful techniques for tying off a limb or torso.

Ankle Wrap

One of the most popular pieces we teach, the Ankle Wrap is knee-deep in awesome! It is comfortable even when tied tightly, since it presses the ankles together where they are most padded, rather than side-by-side where ankle bones can rub together. It's also secure, sexy and simple to tie. Plus, it renders your partner helplessly unable to stand up or balance on one foot, especially when tied over boots—a fact that will keep your partner from "bunny-hopping" away from you.

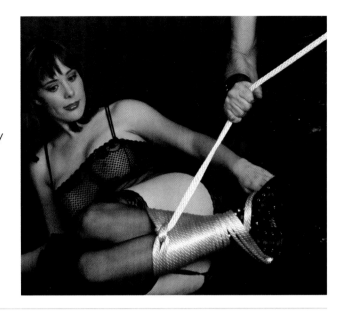

Rope length: 20 to 30 feet (6 – 9m)
Rope diameter: ³⁄₈ to ⁷⁄₁₆ inch (9 – 11mm)

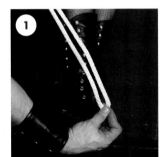

Make a bight in the middle of the rope. Direct this bight toward the bottom of your partner's feet, the toe of the top foot pointing the way.

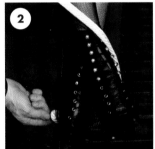

With the working ends held over the top of your partner's crossed ankles, pull the bight under and over to the arch of the bottom foot. Hold the bight in place.

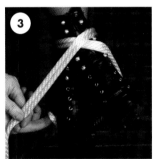

While holding the bight in place with one finger, use your other hand to draw the working ends around the back and over the front of the crossed ankles.

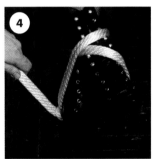

Insert the working ends through the bight.

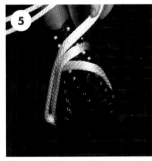

Then pull the working ends up and across the ankles, making sure to keep their rope lines parallel to one another.

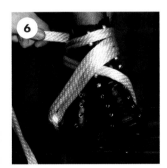

Bring the ropes around the back of the ankles, above and alongside the previous ropes. Keep the ropes tight around the feet and ankles—the firmer the better.

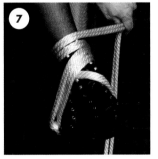

Now simply begin wrapping the ropes around and up the legs, keeping the ropes flat and side-by-side.

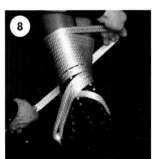

Continue wrapping the ropes up around the legs.

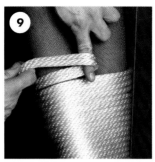

To tie off the piece, use a finger to hold the rope in place while you double back around the back of the calves.

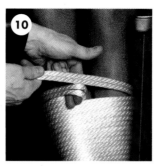

Once the ropes (or working ends) reach the bight you held in place...

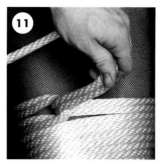

stick them down its loop. Once again, double back your rope ends.

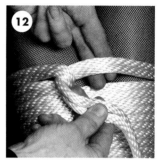

Place a finger or two under the top layer of ropes to hold them up.

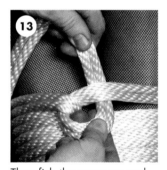

Then fish the ropes up and under this top layer. Leave a small loop open while maintaining tension on the ropes to keep them from sliding.

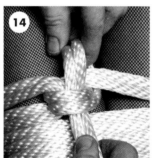

Dive the working ends through this opening...

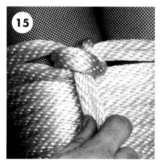

and tighten the knot. Now you can either trim off the excess rope...

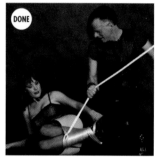

or you can leave the rope ends long, for use in other bondage applications—such as the Ankle Wrap Game!

Ankle Wrap Game

A common question we're asked is, "What do you do once your partner is tied?" Our thoughts are typically, "What don't you do?" Still, we understand imaginations sometimes need a nudge, so here's a fun game you can play once your partner's ankles are bound in an Ankle Wrap. Called the Ankle Wrap Game, the object is not to fall over! Sounds easy? Try doing it when your arms are tied behind your back and your partner is pulling your feet up, moving your center of gravity slightly forward!

Rope length: 30 feet (9m)
Rope diameter: ³/₈ to ⁷/₁₆ inch (9 – 11mm)

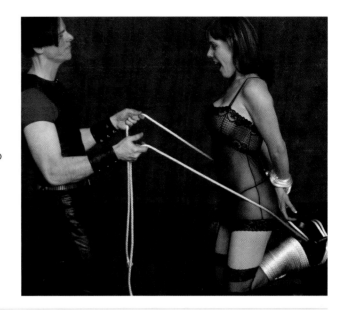

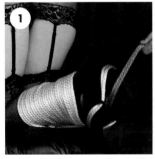

Tie the ankles using the Ankle Wrap, leaving about 5 feet (1.5m) of long rope after it's secure. You may want to provide a pillow for your partner to kneel on for comfort.

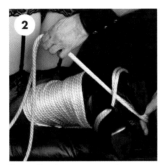

Pass the long ropes down the shins and pull them out between the crossed feet.

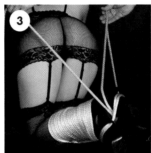

Separate the ropes so one goes around each side of your partner's body.

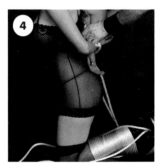

Using a separate piece of rope, tie your partner's wrists behind the back using the Basic Wrap. Make the wrap as long or short as needed for your partner's comfort.

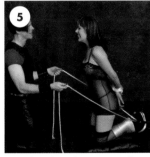

Kneel a shot distance in front of your partner and take a rope in each hand. Say, "Now we're going to play a game. The name of the game is 'Don't fall over.'"

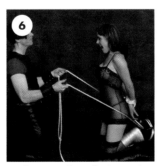

"What are the rules? Don't fall over!" Now slowly pull the ropes, lifting your partner's feet. As you tug on the ropes, your partner's center of gravity shifts forward...

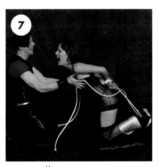

eventually causing your partner to fall forward into your hands, chest or lap. (Oh, and please be sure to actually catch your partner).

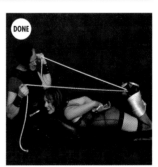

There's no easier way to put your partner in the lap of luxury, for some tender head petting...or other head-related activities.

Basic Wrap

This is one of the most versatile and useful bondage techniques you will ever use! It's great for tying wrists to wrists and for other limb-to-limb applications. It can also be used to tie wrists or ankles to various fixtures or furniture parts, such as the post of a bed or the leg of a chair. The section following this will show you even more techniques, like how to use the wrap as a great handhold for controlling your partner.

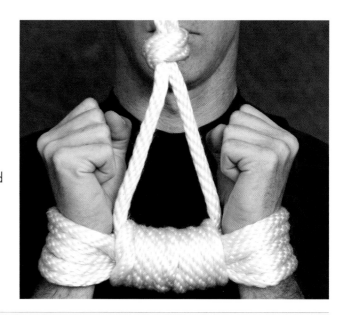

Rope length: 25 feet (8m)
Rope diameter: ¼ to ⁷⁄₁₆ inch (6 – 11mm)

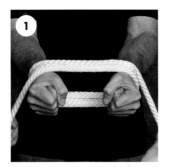

With your partner's limbs apart by the distance of about two fists, lay the middle of your rope over both limbs and wind two wraps toward the elbows, then two toward the fists.

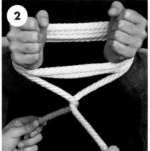

This totals five wraps across. If you're using thinner rope than ⅜ inch (9mm) use additional wraps to distribute the pressure. On the under side, cross the front and back ropes.

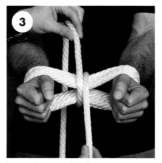

Now bring the front rope over the back side and the back rope over the front side of the wraps.

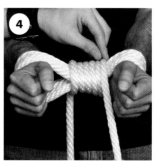

Wind the right rope from the middle toward the limb on your right. Stop winding when you reach a distance of about one finger separation between the skin and the winding.

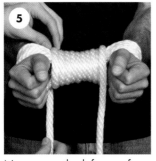

Now wrap the left rope from the middle to the limb on your left. Ideally, you should wind an equal number of wraps on each side of the middle where the ropes crossed.

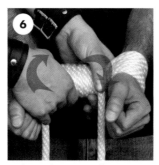

Tighten the wraps by using both hands to twist them in opposite directions, or in the direction each rope was wound.

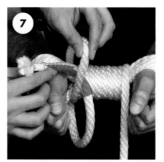

Tie off the wrap by lifting the last loop of the winding and bringing the end of the rope through this loop, passing it from the inside to the outside.

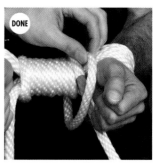

Repeat the tie-off on the other wrist. Secure both finishing knots by pulling on the ends of the ropes. Like we say in the bondage business, "That's a wrap!"

Basic Wrap Applications

Tying someone using the Basic Wrap is just the beginning of the fun. The wrap itself can be used to control your partner in a number of creative and innovative ways. For instance, the following shows a handful of techniques you can use to handle your partner when the Basic Wrap is applied to the wrists.

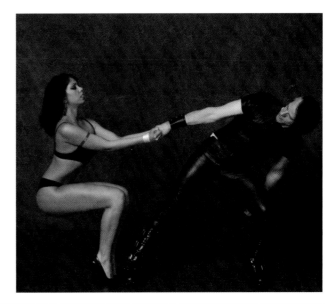

Rope length: 25 feet (8m)
Rope diameter: ¼ to ⁷/₁₆ inch (6 – 11mm)

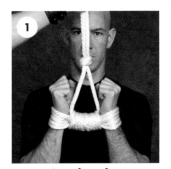

Arms Overhead
Tying both ropes together enables you to lead your partner around or raise the ropes up and through an eyebolt in the ceiling to secure both arms overhead.

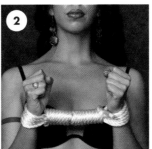

Even without the leading ropes, the basic wrap provides great leverage and a great handhold you can use to control your partner's position.

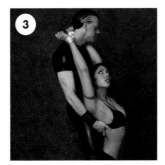

Back Stretch (from Behind)
By placing the wrapped wrists behind your neck, you can immobilize and stretch your partner while your hands remain free to play with your partner's upper body.

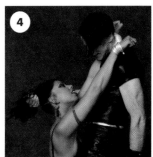

Back Stretch (from Front)
Standing in front, with your kneeling partner's head at your waist level and the wrap behind your neck, opens up a whole other range of fun and control!

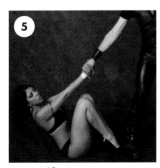

Easy Lift Up
Use the wrap to lift up your partner with amazing ease. With your partner's knees bent and feet together, place the side of your foot against his or her toes.

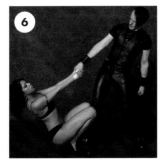

Keep your arm straight and lean to your side. This uses Archimedes' principle of the lever to expend less effort when lifting a body, even one that outweighs you.

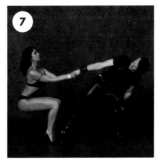

Bend the knee farthest from your partner to maximize the effect of your weight while leaning away and down. With your foot acting like a fulcrum...

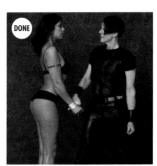

and your straight arm acting like a crane, gently lift up your partner to a standing position.

Prone Tie

This extension of the Basic Wrap is the best method for tying your partner into a prone position—a position that's sublimely submissive. Relatively easy to tie, yet nearly impossible to escape, the piece is a super way to prepare your special someone for spanking, flogging or sex. Due to the stability of the piece, your partner can be rolled onto the side or even onto the back, opening up even more creative options and possibilities.

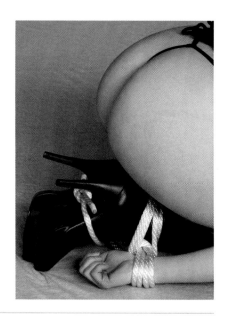

Rope length: 30 feet (9m)
Rope diameter: ³⁄₈ to ⁷⁄₁₆ inch (9 – 11mm)

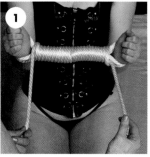

1 Start with a Basic Wrap on the wrists.

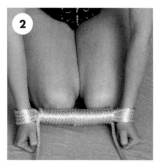

2 The wrap must be tied wide enough to allow the wrists to pass around the outside of your partner's knees and thighs. Have your partner kneel just behind the wrist wrap.

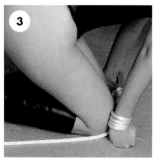

3 Place a pillow in front of the knees, to support and cushion your partner's head and neck for the steps that follow.

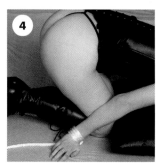

4 Help guide your partner forward until both knees pass over the wrap and the wrists are beside the shins. Make sure your pillow is in place before initiating this step.

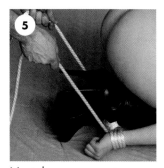

5 Next, have your partner point his or her toes to the floor. Grab the loose ropes leading from the wrists and position the wrap directly under the ankles.

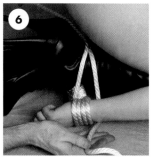

6 Cross both ropes behind the ankles.

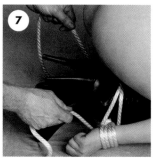

7 Pull the right-hand rope under the wrist wrap, from the front to the back.

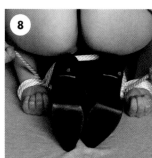

8 Wind the left-hand rope forward under the wrist wrap and pull it up between the left forearm and ankle. Ensure each rope pulls from opposite sides of the wrist wrap.

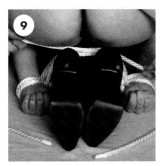

Cross the ropes again across both ankles.

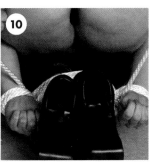

Wind each rope around the wrist wrap in the opposite direction, so they come up from opposite sides of the wrap (front and back).

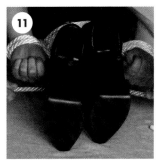

Bring the ropes across both ankles again, but this time cross them underneath the feet.

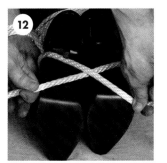

Bring the ropes up over the sides of the feet and cross them under the arch of the heels.

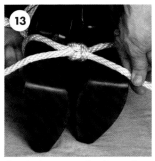

Cinch the ropes firmly and tie them off with a Square Knot.

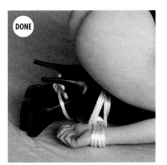

Now relax and enjoy the fant-ass-tic presentation.

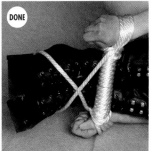

Here's how the ropes look, crossed in the front. Rolled onto the side, your partner remains equally prone to your enjoyment.

Decorative Applications

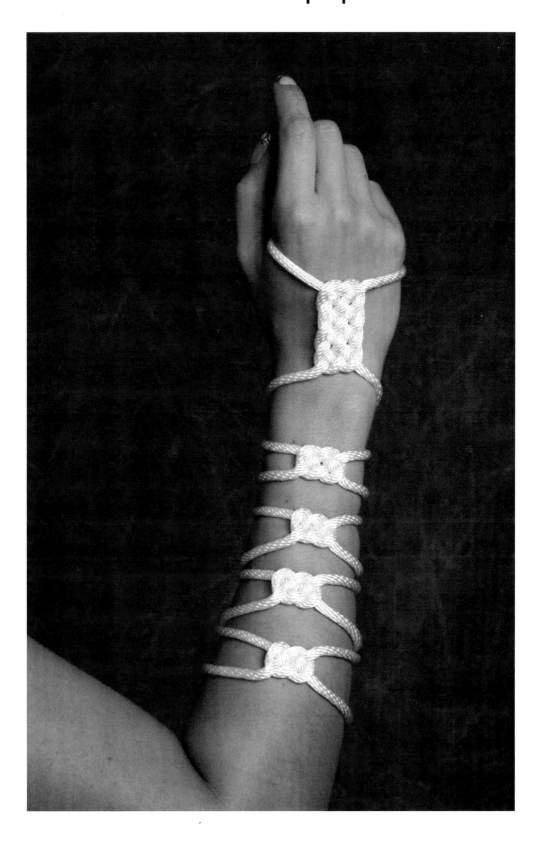

Rope Belt and Buckle

The Rope Belt and Buckle was a serendipitous discovery that resulted from tying a Prosperity Knot with a $7/16$ inch (11mm) rope. At the moment of the knot's completion, we realized its similarity to the look of a large buckle and honed the piece. A fun addition to any outfit, it's bound to get attention and make you look hip—or at least make people look at your hips!

Rope length: 10 to 15 feet (3 – 5m)
Rope diameter: $3/8$ to $7/16$ inch (9 – 11mm)

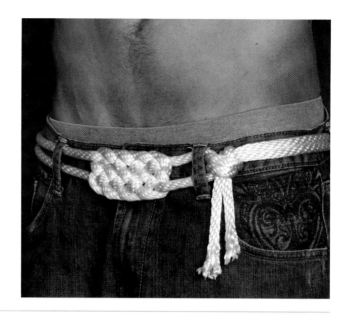

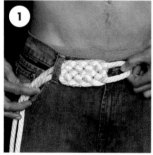

Begin by tying a Prosperity Knot a fist distance down from the middle of your rope. Then, tuck the two working ends of rope through the first belt loop.

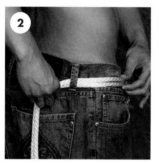

Continue passing the working ends around...

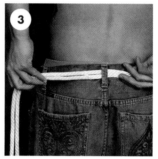

through all the...

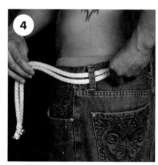

remaining belt loops...

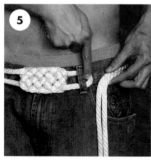

until you return to the looped side of the Prosperity Knot.

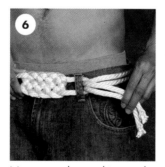

Now pass the working ends through the back of the loop.

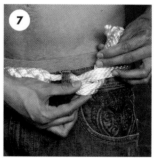

Pull the rope to the desired tightness while tucking the working ends under the belt, over the top and...

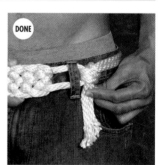

through the loop you created. Cinch the rope down to size and you're ready for a night on the town with the guys.

Rigger Gauntlets

Rigger Gauntlets are essentially a series of half hitches resulting in an elegant and attractive spiral design along the forearm. Relatively easy to tie on one's self, the gauntlets are a great way to "fly your flag" at a play party, or show your rope skills when a partner isn't readily available. Still, whatever your reason for tying the gauntlets, on yourself or another, the person wearing them will be sure to get attention!

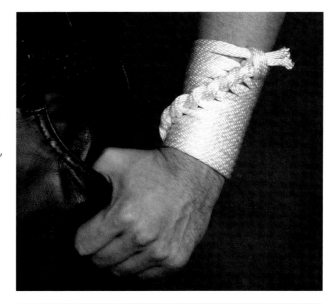

Rope length: 20 to 30 feet (6 – 9m)
Rope diameter: ¼ inch (6mm)

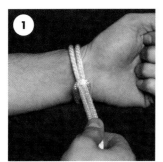

Start off by making a bight at the middle of your rope, then sliding the working ends of rope through the bight's end. Slide this loop around your wrist.

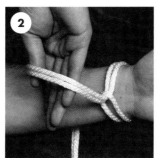

Drop the working ends behind your wrist.

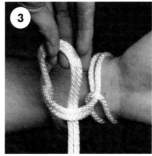

Slide a loop back toward the front of your wrist and pinch the dangling working ends between your forefinger and thumb.

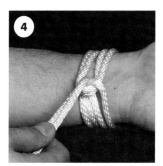

Pull the working ends through this loop.

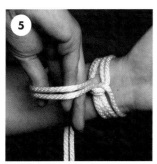

The second verse is the same as the first. Drop the working ends of rope behind your wrist, again.

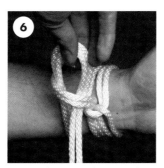

Slide a loop back toward the front of your wrist. Pinch the dangling working ends between your forefinger and thumb...

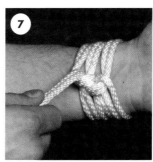

and pull the working ends through this loop.

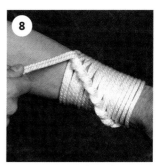

Repeat Steps 2 though 7 until approximately 10 inches of working end (25cm) remain atop your forearm.

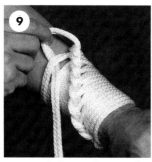

Now tuck the working ends over and under the top two rows of rope.

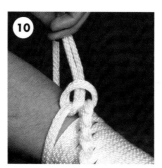

Then tuck the working ends through this loop...

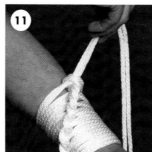

and pull them firmly to cinch the piece in place.

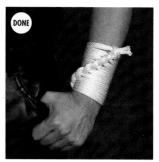

Aside from providing extra support around the wrists, the finished gauntlets let the world know you're game for a good time!

Double Coin Shirt

This piece and the one that follows are the best illustration of how knots, especially the Double Coin Knot, can be thought of as "rivets" on a framework of rope. We created the piece in response to a fan's desire to have a decorative top that was easy to tie and built upon knot knowledge she already possessed. After much deliberation, we came up with the following. Best of all, it may be named after coins, but it won't cost you your shirt.

Rope length: Two lengths 30 to 40 feet (9 – 12m)
Rope diameter: 3/8 to 7/16 inch (9 – 11mm)

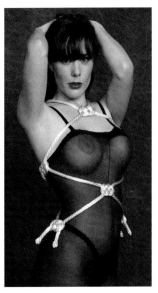
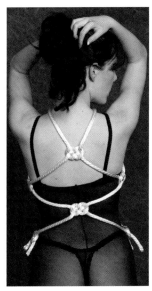

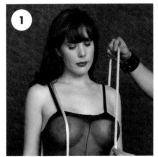

Start with two separate pieces of rope draped over your partner's shoulders.

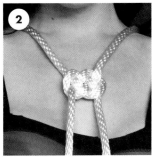

Tie a Double Coin Knot in the middle of your partner's chest, level with the armpits.

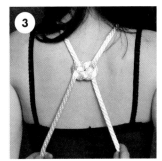

Turn to the back of your partner and tie a Double Coin Knot between the shoulder blades.

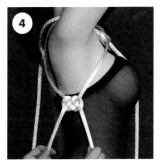

Now split the front and back working ends of rope toward one side of your partner's chest and tie a Double Coin Knot a couple of inches down from the armpit.

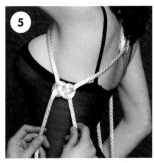

Repeat Step 4 on the other side.

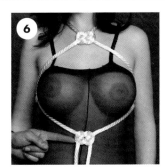

Reunite the front working ends just below your partner's chest and tie another Double Coin Knot.

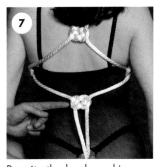

Reunite the back working ends between the middle of your partner's back and the base of the spine and, you guessed it, tie a Double Coin Knot.

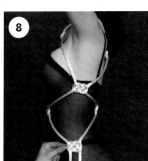

Split the front and back working ends of rope toward one of your partner's hips and tie another Double Coin Knot.

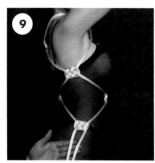

Repeat Step 8 on the other side.

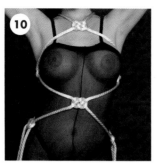

If you have enough rope you could continue on down to your partner's legs to create an attached pair of Rope Stockings, or...

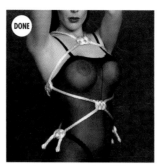

snip the rope ends off for a stand alone top.

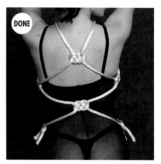

Here's the shirt on your partner's back.

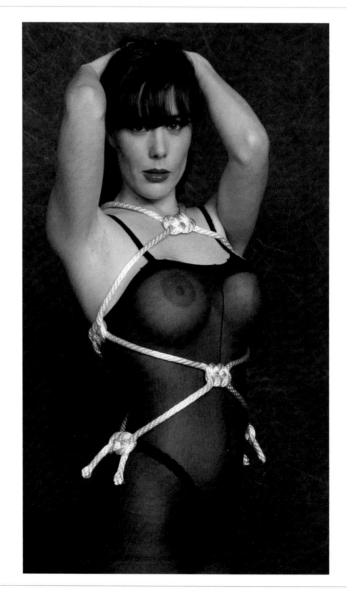

Rope Stockings

The following piece is the logical extension of the Double Coin Shirt. Still, it can also be tied on its own (as shown). Although both the Double Coin Shirt and the Rope Stockings were created to decorate the body, it's important to note their usefulness as connection points for a formidable restraint to a chair or table.

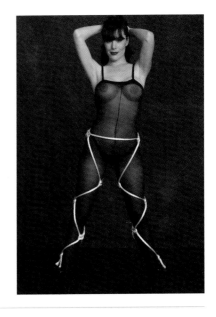

Rope length: Two lengths 30 to 40 feet (9 – 12m)
Rope diameter: ³⁄₈ to ⁷⁄₁₆ inch (9 – 11mm)

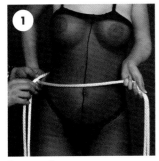

Start with two separate pieces of rope draped over your partner's front and back hips.

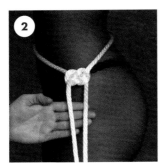

Tie the two ropes together using a Double Coin Knot on each side of your partner's hips. This holds the ropes in place so you can continue tying knots down the leg.

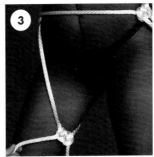

Now, split the working ends of rope from one hip toward the inside of your partner's thigh and tie a Double Coin Knot.

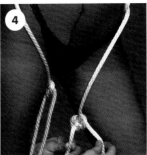

Repeat Step 4 on the other thigh.

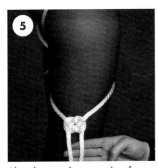

Slip the working ends of rope from an inner thigh toward the outside of your partner's leg and tie another Double Coin Knot.

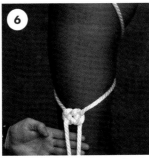

Repeat Step 6 on the other side.

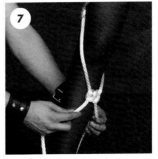

Continue down the legs,

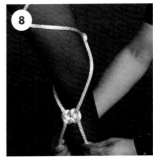

repeating the techniques described in Steps 3 through 6 until...

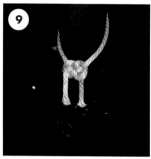

you reach your partner's ankles.

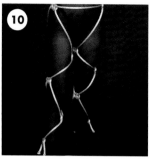

Snip the rope ends off or...

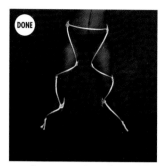

use the excess length to stretch out your partner!

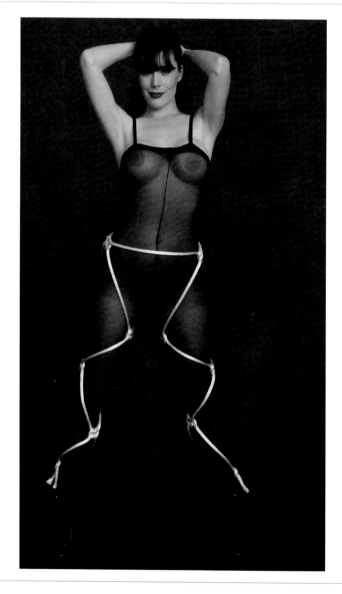

Rope Blindfold

The Rope Blindfold is the product of two strategically placed Prosperity Knots. It's a surprisingly good inhibitor of sight—so much so that anyone blindfolded with the piece should be monitored closely so they don't walk into walls or otherwise hurt themselves. Once the piece is tied, it holds its shape well and can be repeatedly reused without coming undone or loosening. We know you'll agree, it's also quite...eye-catching.

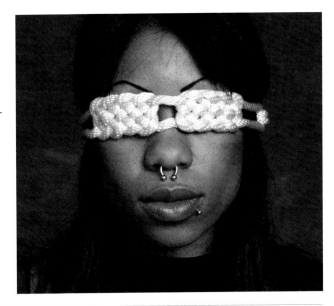

Rope length: 10 to 12 feet (3 – 3.5m)
Rope diameter: ¼ inch (6mm)

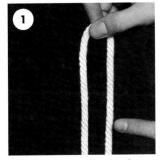

Begin by measuring a distance of 2 inches (5cm) down from the middle of your rope.

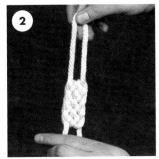

Tie a Prosperity Knot at the base of the measured distance, such that the top of the knot is 2 inches (5cm) from the middle of your rope.

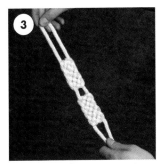

Tie a second Prosperity Knot 1 inch (2.5cm) below the base of the first Prosperity Knot.

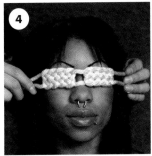

Carefully place the blindfold over the eyes of your partner.

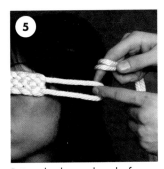

Bring the looped end of rope back past your partner's ear, wrapping the two working ends around the other side of the head.

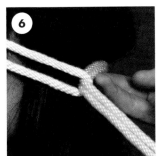

Tuck the working ends underneath and out the looped end of rope.

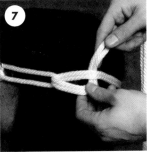

Now tuck the working ends underneath the horizontal ropes...

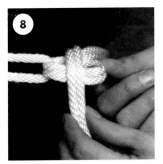

over the small loop created...

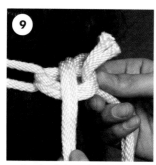

under and then back up through the small loop you just created.

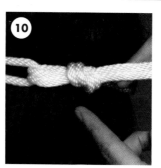

Pulling the working ends firmly will hold the piece in place.

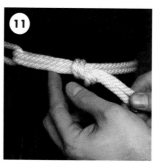

Sliding the knot along the horizontal ropes adjusts the piece to your partner's comfort.

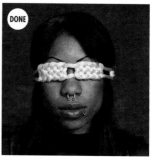

Now wave your hands and stick out your tongue to check if the blindfold is adjusted properly!

Prosperity Knot Glove

As illustrated throughout this book, the Prosperity Knot can be used in a variety of decorative and functional ties. Here it lends its elegant appearance to the hand for a delicate fingerless wrap or "glove." Capable of being tied short or long, this piece makes a strikingly attractive accessory to a body adorned by a Rope Corset or Harness.

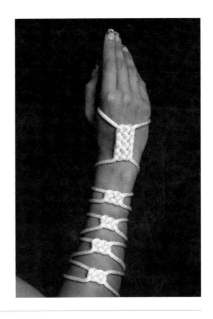

Rope length: 3 to 5 feet (1 – 1.5m)
Rope diameter: ³⁄₁₆ to ¼ inch (3 – 6mm)

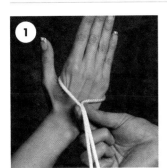

Measure the distance around the palm you are going to tie.

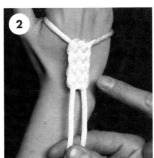

Where the ropes come together at the back of the hand, tie a Prosperity Knot.

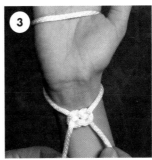

Split the working ends to the front of the wrist and tie a Double Coin Knot.

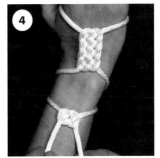

Split the working ends back toward the back of the wrist and tie another Double Coin Knot.

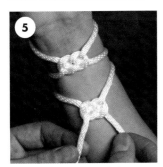

Repeat Steps 3 and 4...

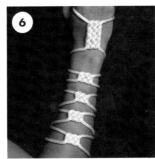

until you've created a forearm length glove...

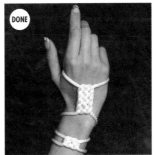

or stop short for a wrist length glove. The choice is yours.

Hair Corset

This hair corset and the rope corsetry and arm gauntlets shown in our first book are applications of kackling, a technique that the *Ashley Book of Knots* states "...is probably the commonest of the knotted forms." Sleek and elegant when tied around the hair, kackling is a convenient way to keep your partner's hair trussed up and out of the way during play. Tying the hair in this way also heightens the sensual connection between partners, especially if the partner being tied enjoys having the hair tugged on or pulled.

Rope length: 25 to 50 feet (8 – 15m)
Rope diameter: ⅛ to ¼ inch (3 – 6mm)

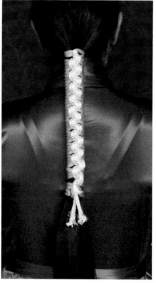 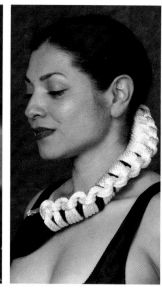

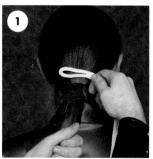

1. Secure a ponytail with an elastic hair tie. Make a bight in the middle of the rope and place this bight around the hair, above the hair tie.

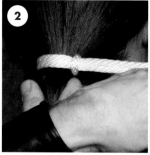

2. Thread both running ends through this bight, positioned above the hair tie, and pull them tightly.

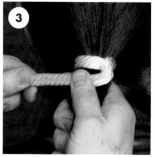

3. With one hand, firmly hold the ponytail and pinch the ropes in one place as you use your other hand to double back the ropes in the opposite direction.

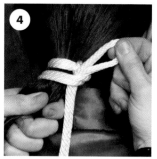

4. Bring the ropes around the back side of the ponytail and up through the opening where the ropes doubled-back.

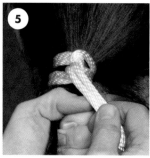

5. Hold the hair firmly again and double back the ropes in the opposite direction.

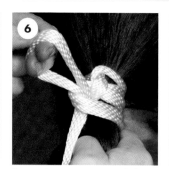

6. Bring the ropes around the back of the ponytail and up through the opening made when the ropes doubled back.

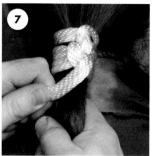

7. Continue alternating this pattern. Make sure all the ropes stay parallel, flat and flush with the previous ropes and that you consistently thread the ropes up.

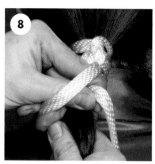

8. Pulling the ropes is easier if you fish your fingers through the opening and pull the ropes back through the loop.

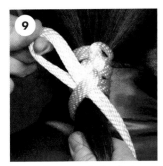

9

Carefully smooth the hair as you wind each layer.

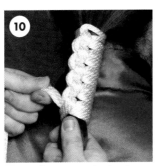

10

Keep alternating the hitches "left and right, up through the bight." Bind the hair as tightly as possible as you do so.

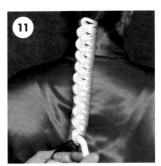

11

Keep the ridge of kackling straight down the center of the ponytail.

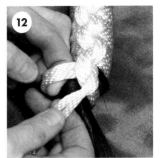

12

When you come near the end of the rope—or the end of the hair—double back one more time, but stick a finger under these ropes, as shown, to make an opening.

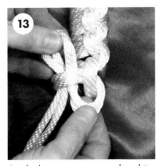

13

Stick the ropes up under this opening and pull them through, while holding another hole open at the bottom of the last double-back.

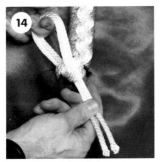

14

Dive the ends of the ropes down through this opening and pull them through to close the loop.

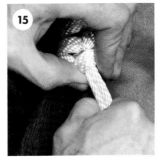

15

Tighten this finishing knot. You can either trim the rope ends or keep them long, to tie the hair into other bondage points.

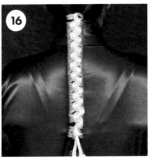

16

The spine-like kackling will turn heads! If working with very fine or slippery hair, you can make the piece more secure by first spraying the ponytail with hair spray.

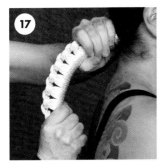

17

If wound tightly enough, you can actually bend the corseted ponytail...

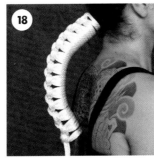

18

and it will maintain its shape in a dramatic curve, downward, to the side or even...

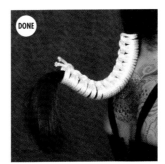

DONE

upward, to create a "hair-rection!"

Rope Collar

One of the most sacred and intimate acts between two partners is the collaring of one partner by another. Considering the significance of such a bond, we created the following piece. Simple yet attractive, the Rope Collar can be pulled against, used in the dynamics of play, or simply worn. The perfect gift for someone special in your life, its offering is made all the more significant by your having made it yourself.

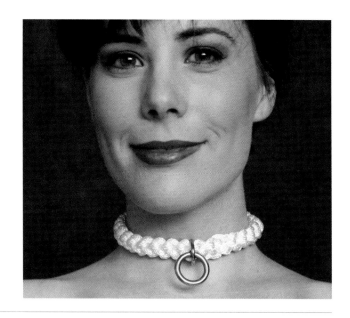

Rope length: 10 feet (3m)
Rope diameter: $3/16$ to $1/4$ inch (3 – 6mm)

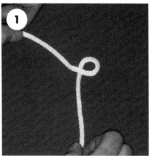

At the middle of your rope, make a loop. Make sure the left-hand rope end is in on top of the loop you created.

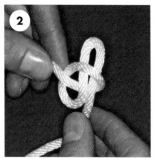

Make a bight with the right working end of rope and push it through the loop you just created.

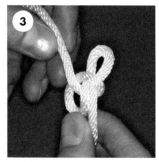

Pull the standing end of rope so that the bight is cinched in place.

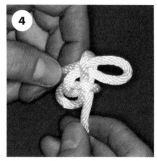

Now make a bight with the standing end of rope (now the working end) and push it through the cinched loop.

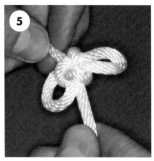

Cinch the second loop in place.

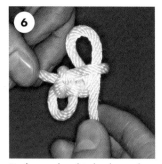

Push another bight through the cinched loop and...

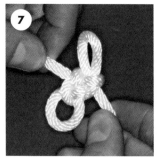

cinch it down.

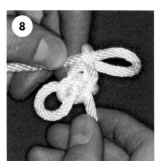

Continue creating bights, pushing them though the loops and...

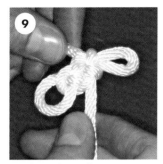

cinching them down.

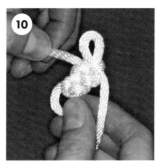

Repeat this back and forth...

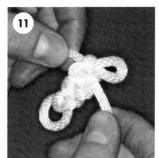

looping and cinching technique, until you reach the desired length of your collar.

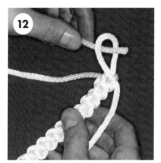

Then, tuck the tip of the working end through the cinched loop,

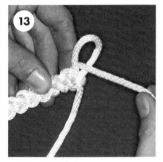

pulling it all the way through, and...

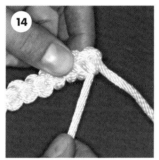

cinching it down.

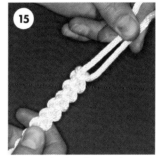

The cinched collar end should look like this.

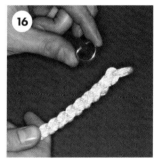

Take an open ½ inch (13mm) D-ring and...

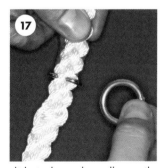

slide it down the collar until you reach its middle.

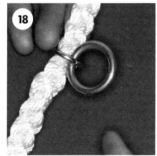

Take a 1 inch (25mm) O-ring and slide it through the opening of the D-ring until you reach the front of the collar.

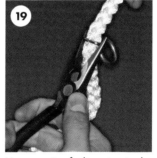

Use a pair of pliers to cinch the D-ring shut.

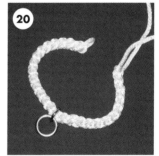

At this point your collar is finished!

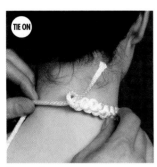

To tie the piece on your partner, lace one of the working ends through the first loop of the collar.

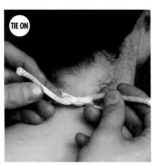

Then, tie the collar off with a square knot.

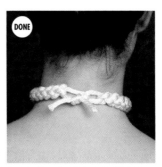

Once finished, trim off the excess rope. Remember to leave enough length for the piece to be retied later.

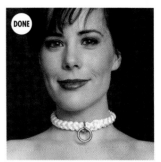

Now go gift your collar to someone special!

Maximum Exposure Ties

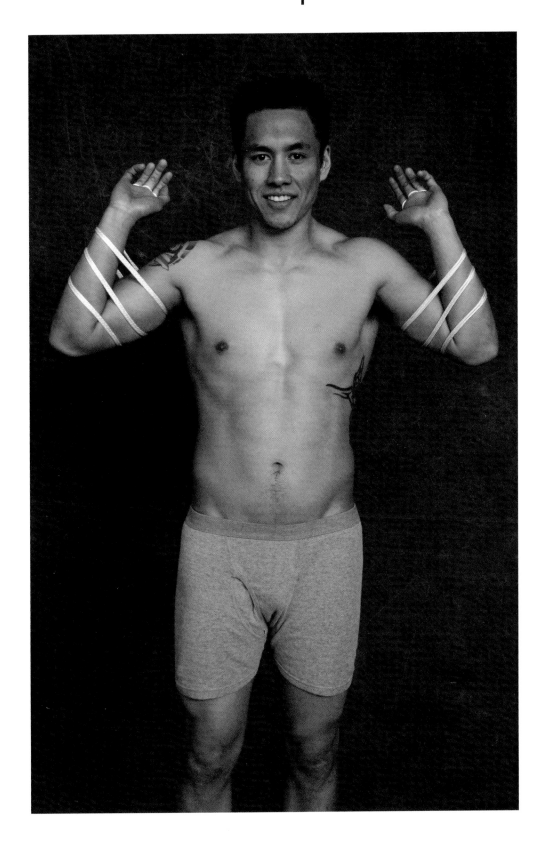

Samurai Tie

The following was one of the first pieces we taught publicly. Based upon a *Hojojutsu* tie (a technique used in feudal Japan to restrain prisoners with rope), we elaborated upon it to incorporate our unique brand of engineering and esthetic. As an aside, there are a variety of Hojojutsu ties to explore and learn, each denoting the prisoners' military rank, class of society or their particular offense. So, if you want to expand your exploration of rope bondage beyond this book, know that there are other traditions, educators and techniques awaiting your wonder and learning.

Rope length: 20 to 30 feet (6 – 9m)
Rope diameter: ³⁄₈ to ⁷⁄₁₆ inch (9 – 11mm)

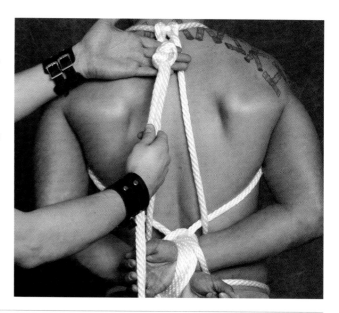

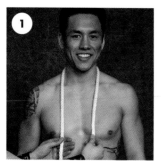

Start with the middle of the rope around the back of your partner's neck.

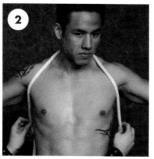

Split the left and right working ends of the rope, tucking them under your partner's left and right armpits, respectively.

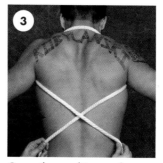

Cross the working ends across the middle of your partner's back.

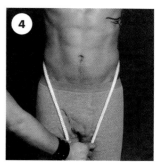

Bring the crossed working ends back to the front over your partner's left and right hips and down between the legs.

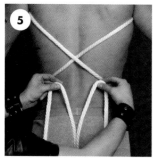

Draw the working ends up your partner's back. Make sure not to "roll" (or cross) your ropes.

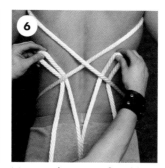

Now, tuck a pair of "rabbit ears" (or bights) up and under the lower part of the rope X on your partner's back.

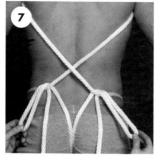

Pull the loops down until the piece firms up.

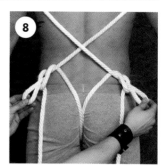

Then, tuck the left and right working ends through the left and right loops, respectively.

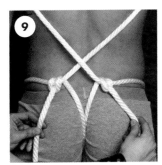

9

You've just created a tie-off point.

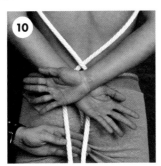

10

To bind the arms, have your partner cross both wrists over your dangling working ends.

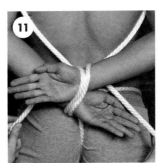

11

Wrap the left and right working ends up and around the wrists.

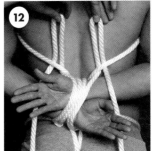

12

Then, tuck the left and right working ends under the top part of the X on your partner's back and pull through.

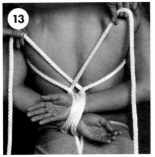

13

Cross the working ends and...

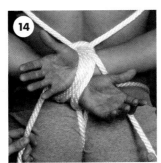

14

bring them down again, splitting them between the front and back of your partner's wrists.

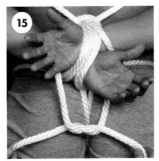

15

Tie an overhand knot at the base of the wrists, and...

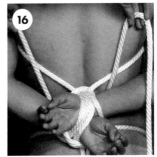

16

then draw the working ends up, between the front and the back of your partner's wrists until you reach the neckline.

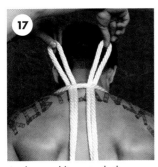

17

At the neckline, tuck the working ends under and...

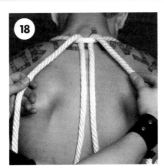

18

pull the working ends all the way through the rope along the neckline.

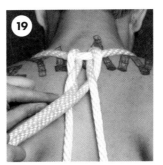

19

Pull the left and right working ends down and around the outside of the parallel ropes lined up with the spine.

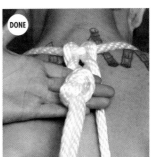

DONE

Finish the piece by tying a double overhand knot.

Cinching Ball Tie

As the name implies, the Cinching Ball Tie curls a person into a ball of sorts, opening her up to a number of playful options. When tied up in this manner and rolled forward, your partner becomes fully exposed and accessible for spanking and flogging, or highly receptive for just about any input (so to speak). The piece also remains easy to remove once you're done having a ball together.

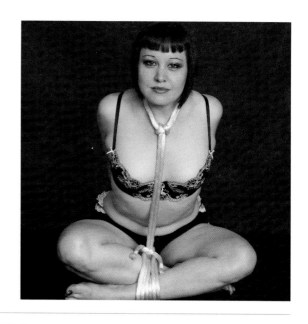

Rope length: 20 to 30 feet (6 – 9m)
Rope diameter: ³/₈ to ⁷/₁₆ inch (9 – 11mm)

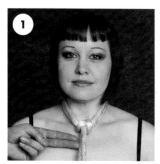

Start by tying a Rope Shackle around your partner's neck. The working ends of the shackle should come forward toward your partner's legs.

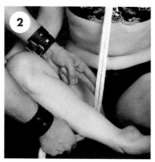

Have you partner cross one ankle over the working ends of rope.

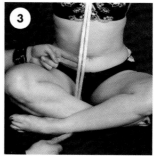

Then have your partner cross the other ankle over the working ends.

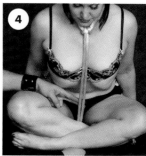

Pull the working ends forward so that your partner's neck is a comfortable distance forward, but not so far forward that it strains the neck or back.

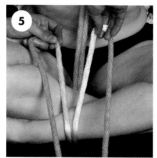

Wrap the left and right working ends of rope...

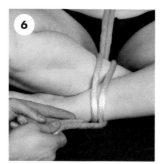

around the ankles. Make sure to split the working ends on either side of the extended rope.

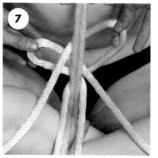

Now cross the left and right working ends behind the point where the extended rope connects to the ankles.

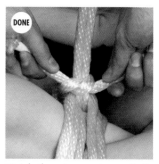

Finish the piece using a Split Square Knot.

Consequence Tie

Simply put, the following tie gently slides rope over the sex parts as a "consequence" for straightening the legs or rocking back and forth. Discovered serendipitously while playing with a feisty partner, the piece is the innovative combination of a Shackle Tie and a Double Slipknot. Still, the real star of the show is the rope between these two foundation ties. Circuitously woven from the ankles to the hips and then between the legs, the rope creates a simple machine that generates tantalizing pleasure and self-inflicted fun!

Rope length: 20 feet (6m)
Rope diameter: ³⁄₈ to ⁷⁄₁₆ inch (9 – 11mm)

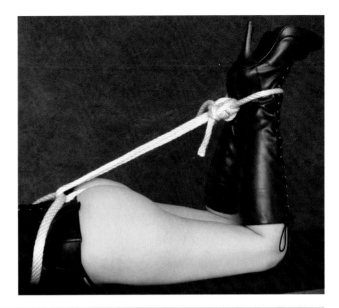

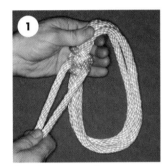

Start by tying a Rope Shackle, either by pre-making it in your hand large enough to place over the waist, or by tying directly around the waist.

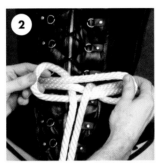

Adjust the tightness of the shackle around the waist by first pulling on the sides of the knot to allow the shackle loops to slip and cinch tighter...

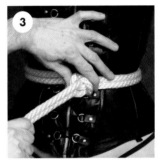

and then retightening the knot by pulling on the rope ends.

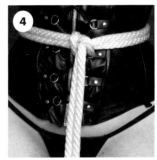

Center it on the waist.

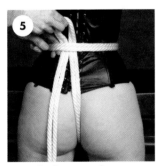

Bring both ropes down between the legs, then up to the waist and under the wraps of the shackle.

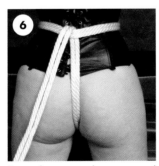

Drop the ropes down toward the feet.

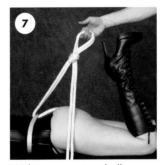

With your partner belly-down on the floor, with knees bent about 45 degrees, mark the distance where the working ends of the rope meet the ankles.

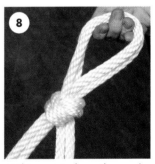

At this point along the working ends, tie a Double Slipknot.

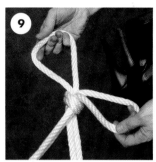

Spread the loops of the Double Slipknot.

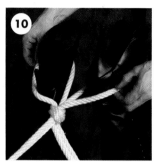

Bend the knees and place each loop over its respective ankle.

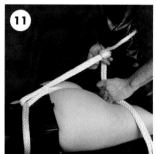

Tighten the Double Slipknot around the ankles.

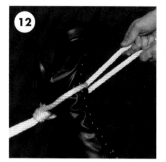

Bring the rope ends under the knot, between the ankles...

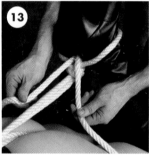

and then back over the knot.

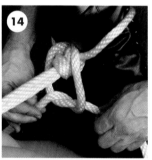

Tie a Split Square Knot starting on the bottom of the rope branching off the Double Slip Knot...

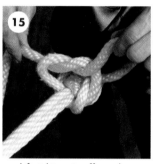

and finishing it off on the top.

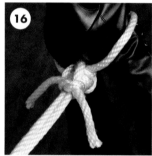

Tighten the knot and trim the excess rope.

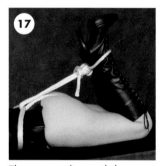

The wearer lies with knees bent and ankles close to the butt and the rope between the legs.

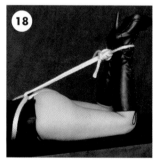

If the ropes are struggled against (or the legs are straightened), the "machine" is set into motion and stimulation begins.

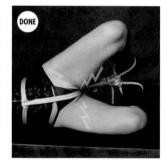

Here's how it looks lying on the side. The cool part is that it is the wearer who controls the intensity of the stimulation.

T-Back

An extension of the Basic Wrap, this solid piece of bondage makes a struggle-proof upper arm restraint. Its comfortable fit and elegant engineering create an easy access grip for handling and maneuvering your partner from behind, even when the piece is covered by a loose jacket or blouse—hint, hint. The piece also assists in keeping the chest out and arms back during posture training play.

Rope length: 20 to 30 feet (6 – 9m)
Rope diameter: 3/8 to 7/16 inch (9 – 11mm)

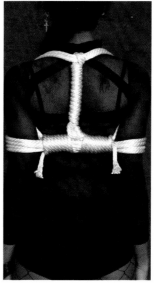
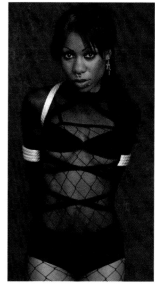

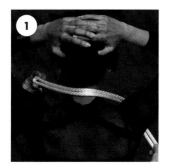

1 Make a bight in the middle of the rope. Draw this bight under the right armpit and around the back of the neck...

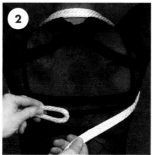

2 then in front and under the left armpit. The bight and the working ends of rope should meet at the center of the back.

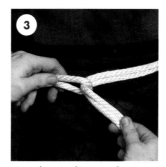

3 Pass the working ends through the bight, like so.

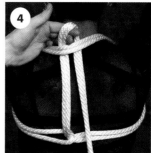

4 Bring the working ends of rope up to the neckline and tuck them under and over the ropes that pass around the back of the neck.

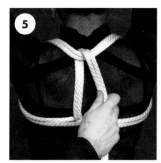

5 Bring the working ends down. Take a moment to adjust the tension of the ropes around the body, sliding them as needed to reduce slack and center the bight on the spine.

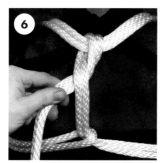

6 Now start wrapping the working ends around the back of the vertical ropes, from right to left.

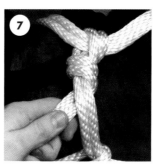

7 Continue winding the working ends all the way down the vertical ropes.

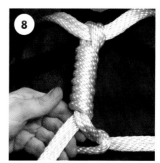

8 Keep the ropes parallel to one another as you lay them side by side. Stop winding once you reach the bight.

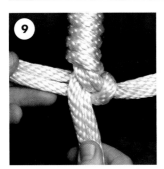

Drop the working ends of the rope over the left side of the bight...

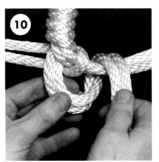

then under, behind and over the horizontal ropes to the left of the bight. As you do so, maintain an open loop to receive the ropes when they come over the top.

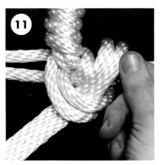

Thread the working ends down through the open loop.

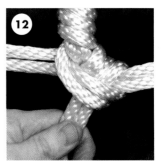

Secure this stage of the piece by pulling firmly on the working ends.

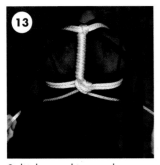

Split the working ends apart, wrapping each around your partner's left and right bicep, respectively.

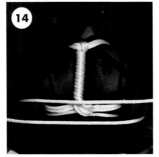

Continue wrapping each working end around your partner's arms. Make sure both remain parallel to one another.

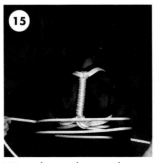

Wrap the working ends around your partner's left and right biceps again.

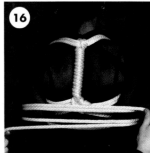

Continue wrapping around your partner's arms until the four winds are complete and the left and right working ends reach the bottom of the T-Back, behind the winds.

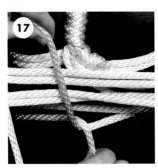

When both working ends are behind the horizontal winds, cross them.

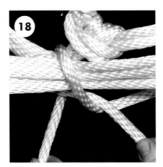

Wind the left working end of rope over the top and around the back of ALL the ropes left of your partner's spine (including the ropes that led to the bight).

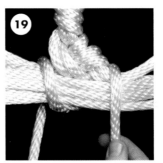

Wind the right working end under and around the front of ALL the ropes on the right side of your partner's spine, just as you did with the left working end.

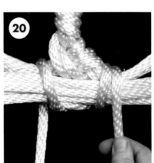

Begin winding the right rope around all the horizontal ropes on the right side.

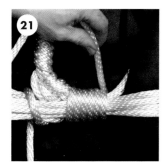

21

Keep all the winds parallel to one another.

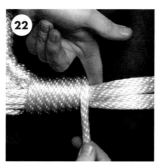

22

Stop winding when you reach a distance of one finger width between the winding and the arm. This helps maintain proper circulation through the arm's brachial artery.

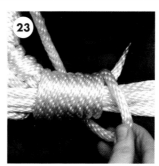

23

Tie off the winding by lifting the last coil of rope to create an open loop...

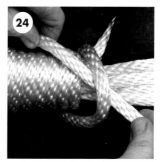

24

and tucking the right working end through the loop, from the inside to the outside. This finish is the same one used to tie off the Basic Wrap.

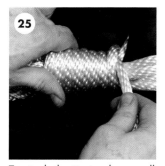

25

To cinch the tie in place, pull on the working end. Make sure to keep one finger space between the rope and the arm.

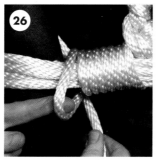

26

Repeat Steps 20 through 22 on the left side, lifting the last coil of rope...

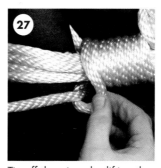

27

Tie off the piece by lifting the last winding to create a loop, then tucking the working end through this loop (just as you did on the right side).

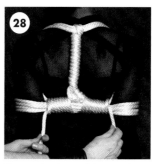

28

Tug on both working ends to assure the piece is firmly in place.

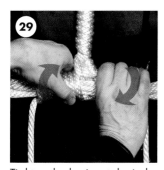

29

Tighten the horizontal windings by twisting them in opposite directions—in the same direction each was wound.

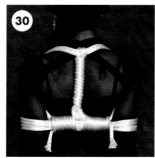

30

At this point, you can cut off the excess rope or use what rope remains to tie your partner's wrists.

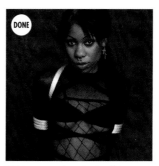

DONE

Wrists can be tied off in front of or behind your partner's body—your choice.

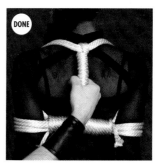

DONE

Whichever you choose, you will be able to "handle" it!

Dildo Strap-On Harness

If you're looking for a great time with a dildo, now you can really tie one on—even if you don't own a fancy adjustable leather strap-on harness. Utilizing the center opening of the Box Knot, this piece holds just about any flanged (wide-based) dildo firmly in place. Meanwhile, the working ends of the rope branching off the Box Knot make for "straps" that adjust to the shape of your body.

Rope length: 25 feet (7m)
Rope diameter: ¼ inch (6mm)

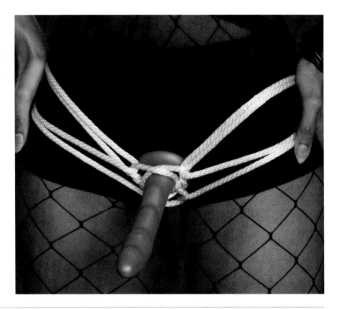

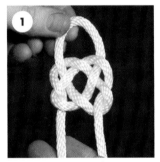

1 Tie a Box Knot at the very middle of your rope. Leave a small loop at the top.

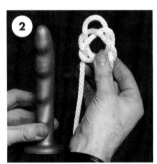

2 Spread the center opening of the Box Knot just wide enough to accept the diameter of the dildo.

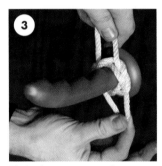

3 Slide the Box Knot down to the hilt of the flanged dildo. Keep the loop of the Box Knot on the "underside" of the dildo.

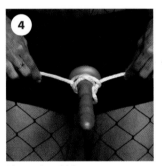

4 Place the dildo on your pubic area at the most anatomically appropriate (or comfortable) position. Bring the ropes around your lower hips.

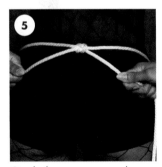

5 Cinch the ropes securely around your hips and tie them with a Square Knot.

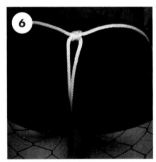

6 Pass the ends of the ropes down under your butt...

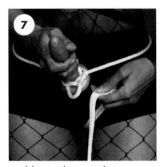

7 and bring them up between your legs, keeping them together without twisting them, so as not to get your panties in a bunch. (Then again, why even wear panties?)

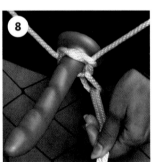

8 Pass these ropes through the loop at the bottom of the Box Knot.

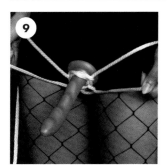

Part the ropes and bring one around each side of your pelvis, horizontally across the top of your thighs.

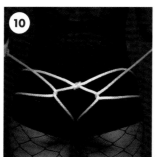

Pull each rope through the opening in the rope at the back below the Square Knot. Pull each rope firmly as you bring it around the upper hip on each side...

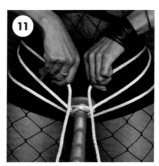

and back to the front, above all previous ropes.

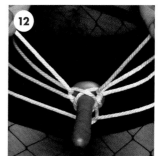

Thread each rope through its nearest loop on the upper corner of the Box Knot. Keep pulling firmly as you pass them back around your upper hips.

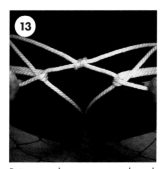

Bring each rope around and down to the opening below the Square Knot and pull it outward toward the side.

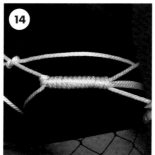

While pulling the ropes to keep the piece as taut as possible, begin winding each rope around the three lower lines across the butt.

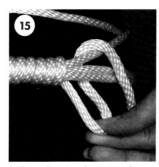

When the winding reaches near the side of the hip, make a small loop (or rabbit ear).

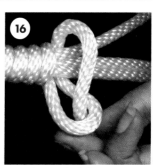

Pass the end of the rope through the opening...

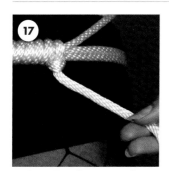

and cinch it down to collapse the loop, thus tying off the piece.

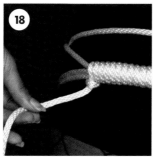

Do the same winding and tying off with the rope on the other side.

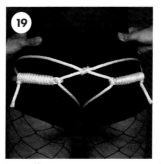

Cut off any excess rope.

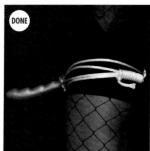

Adjust the angle and position of your dildo. Fasten your harness and enjoy the ride.

Head Cage

Head ties nearly always come out looking sloppy. This is more often the case because the roundness of the head is a challenge to most, leading to guesswork and over-tying. With these frustrations in mind, we created the Head Cage, a tie that provides the framework for a clean and functional head tie. Once completed, this piece can be used to control the head, assist in the functionality of a gag or simply act as a decorative harness for a high-impact look that really turns heads.

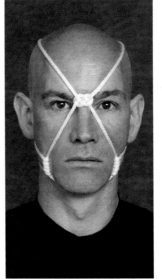
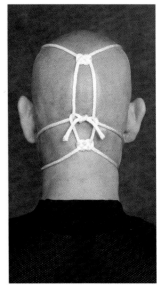

Rope length: 10 to 12 feet (3 – 3.5m)
Rope diameter: ¼ inch (6mm)

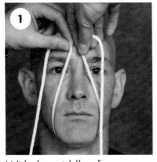

With the middle of your rope under your partner's chin, bring both working ends up from the chin to the bridge of the nose and note that distance.

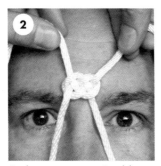

At this point, tie a Double Coin Knot. Make sure to maintain the knot's flatness. Tighten it snugly.

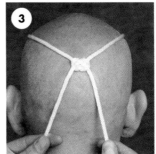

Measure the distance from the bridge of your partner's nose to the crown of the head. At this point, tie another Double Coin Knot.

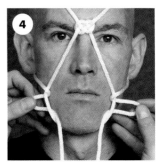

Split the working ends under the ears, back toward the level of your partner's mouth.

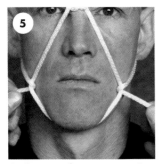

At the top of your partner's mouth, begin winding the left and right working ends over the left and right parallel ropes…

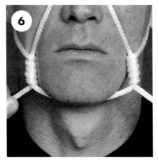

until the winds reach the space just above the chin.

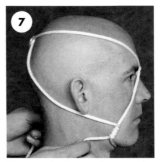

Now, split the working ends back toward the base of the neck.

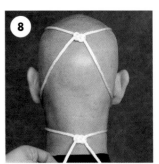

At the base of the neck, tie another Double Coin Knot.

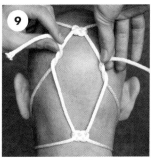

9 Then bring the left and right working ends up and over the left and right ropes above.

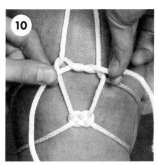

10 Cross the working ends, pulling them snug, and...

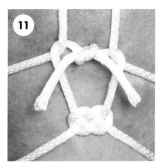

11 fix the piece in place with a snug Square Knot.

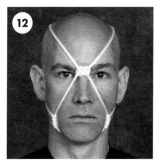

12 The finished piece results in...

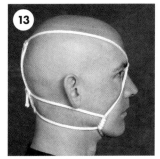

13 a clean looking, yet...

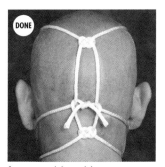

DONE functional head harness.

Claw

This deceptively simple piece can be used to inhibit the movement of the wrists and hands. Called the Claw, it functionally restricts a person's lower arms while allowing the use of the shoulders. Massively frustrating for the person tied, the piece can also be used to inhibit the ability to push off the floor or keep someone from pressing closer. The only caveat to the use of this piece is that it should be avoided by persons with carpal tunnel syndrome or tendonitis of the wrists.

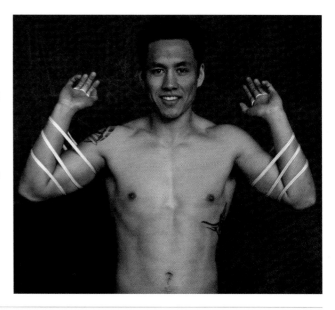

Rope length: 10 to 12 feet (3 – 3.5m)
Rope diameter: ¼ inch (6mm)

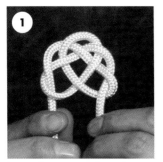

Begin by tying a Box Knot at the middle point of your rope.

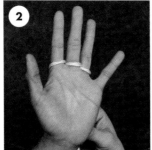

Separate the side and middle loops and slide them over your partner's index, middle and ring finger. The loops should not restrict circulation. If they do, loosen them!

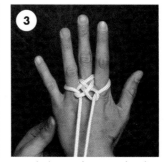

Gently bring the wrist back so that the back of the fingers are about three inches (8cm) from the top of the shoulder. (Vary depending on your partner's flexibility.)

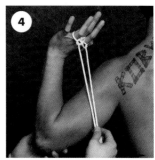

Now wrap the working ends of rope under the tricep...

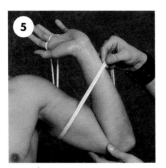

over the wrist...

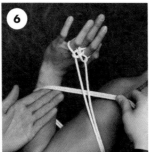

then underneath the parallel ropes branching off the fingers.

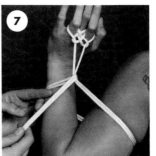

Bight the working ends back over the wrist and...

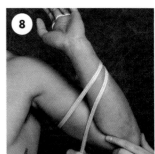

underneath the tricep again. Leave a two finger space between the first wrap and the second.

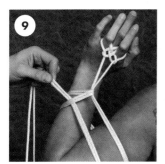

9 Now tuck the working ends underneath the bight above. The wraps do not have to be "rock tight" for the piece to hold. Adjust the tightness of the wraps to your partner's limits.

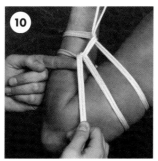

10 Bight the working ends back under the tricep and....

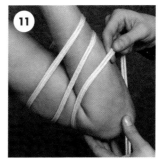

11 over the space before the elbow.

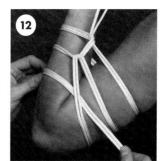

12 Tuck the working ends underneath the next bight in series.

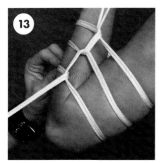

13 Bight the working ends back again.

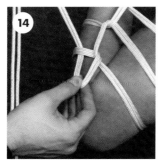

14 This time, tuck the working ends underneath themselves and...

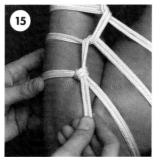

15 then down the loop you created. Pull the working ends firmly to cinch the piece in place.

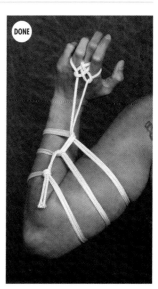

DONE

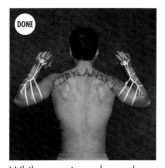

DONE While our piece shows three wraps, feel free to use as many wraps as will fit along the arm and your partner feels comfortable wearing.

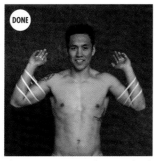

DONE The same tie can be applied to both arms for a more balanced piece that your partner will be up in arms about.

Foot Bender

The Foot Bender is fan service for those who love to restrict the flex of the foot when tickling or "torturing" the feet of their partner. The typical way of isolating the flex of the foot (and restricting movement of the ankles) is to fix the legs in stocks. But stocks prove impractical for most, especially for those who are only casual or occasional players. On the other hand (or rather, the other foot), the Foot Bender provides an impressive restriction of the foot's ability to flex with a whole lot less medieval machinery. (Bonds are often a wiser investment than stocks, anyway.)

Rope length: 10 to 12 feet (3 – 3.5m)
Rope diameter: ¼ inch (6mm)

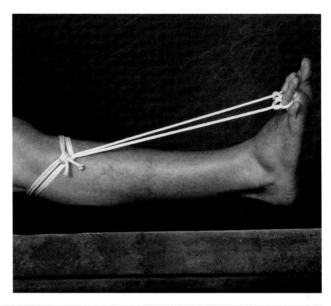

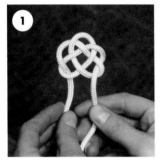

Begin by tying a Box Knot at the middle of your rope.

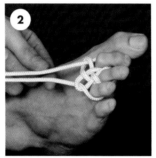

Separate the side and middle loops of the Box Knot and slide them over your partner's index, middle and fourth toes. If the loops restrict circulation, loosen them.

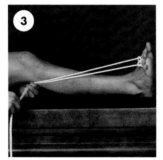

With your partner's foot bent at 90 degrees, bring the working ends of the rope up to the top of the calf. Wrap the working ends of the rope around the back of the calf.

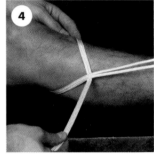

Then, bight the working ends underneath the stretched ropes and...

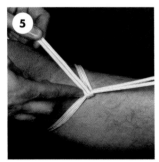

back again around the the calf.

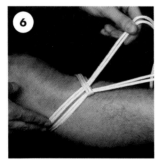

Pass the working ends underneath the bight you created at the calf and...

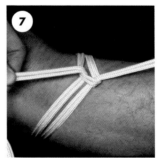

back again.

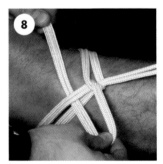

This time, tuck the working ends under themselves and...

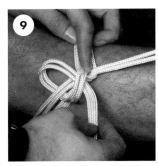 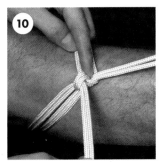 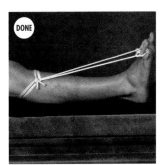

then through the loop you created.

Cinch the working ends in place and...

the tie is complete!

Foot Web

Foot lovers will get a kick out of this foot and ankle binding that is both decorative and functionally restrictive. While holding the ankles side by side, beautiful webbing across the top and between the toes keeps the feet comfortably secured side by side as well. The end product is so stunningly attractive you'll have a hard time choosing whether to move on with your scene or simply sit and stare at your partner's feet!

Rope length: 18 feet (5.5m)
Rope diameter: ⅛ to ¼ inch (3 – 6mm)

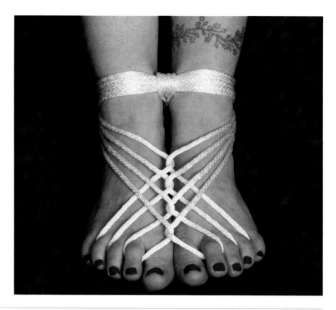

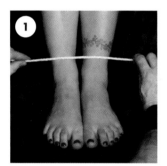

Start with the middle of the rope against the front of your partner's ankles.

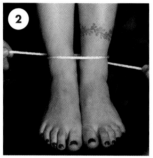

Wrap the working ends once around the back of the ankles

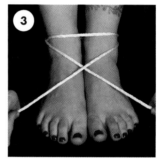

Cross the working ends, right over left, atop the upper part of the feet.

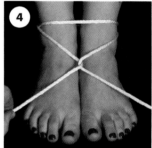

Twist the working ends one half turn, counter-clockwise.

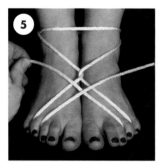

Bring each working end under and around the fourth toe of its respective foot, then cross the ropes, left over right, atop the foot, below the previous twist.

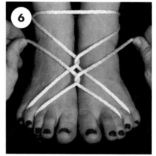

Twist the working ends one half turn, clockwise.

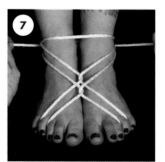

Wrap the working ends once around the back of the ankles...

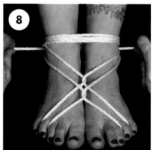

and once around the front of the ankles.

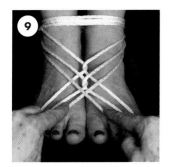

9

Bring the working ends down the foot and cross them, left over right, below the previous twist.

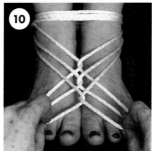

10

Twist the working ends one half turn, counter-clockwise.

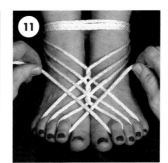

11

Bring each working end under and around the second toe of its respective foot, then cross the ropes, left over right, below the previous twist.

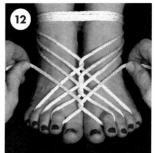

12

Twist the working ends one half turn, clockwise.

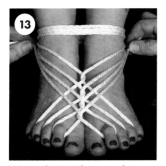

13

Wrap the working ends once around the back and the front of the ankles. Keep the ropes parallel and flat against the skin. Don't wrap the ankles too tightly.

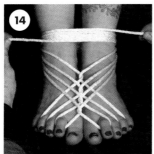

14

Bring the working ends to the back of the ankles and cross them at 90 degrees.

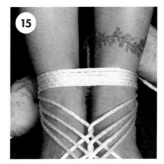

15

Bring the top working end forward, from the back over the top of the wrap, and thread the bottom working end forward from under the bottom of the wrap...

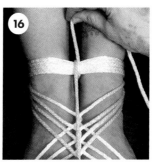

16

and continue wrapping both working ends around to the back...

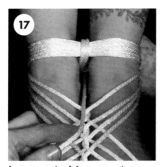

17

for a total of four winds.

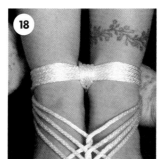

18

Allow a one-finger space between the wound ropes and the ankles...

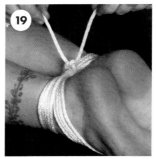

19

then secure the wrap with a square knot at the back of the ankles.

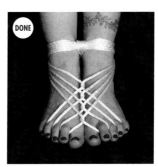

DONE

Now that's some fancy footwork!

Intermediate Harnesses

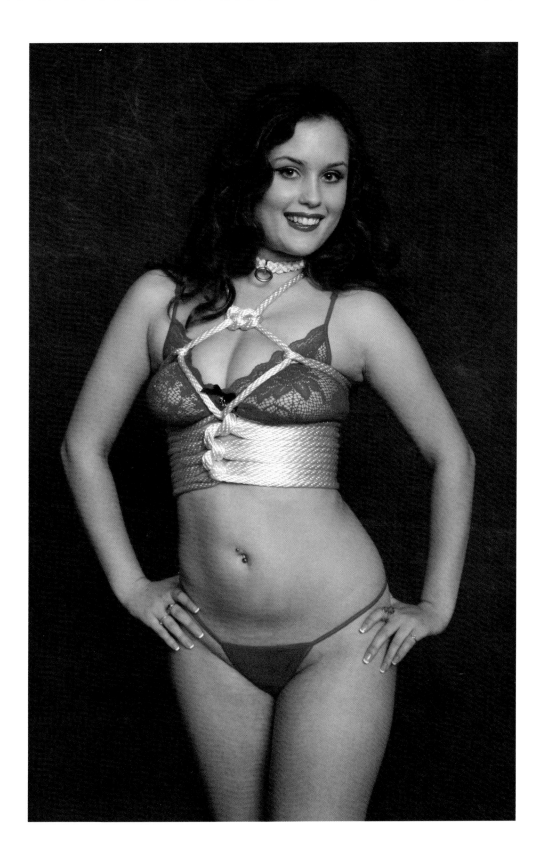

Corselet Harness

A corselet is an undergarment that combines a girdle with a bra. Similar to a traditional corset, corselets were popular from the mid-1910s on through the 1950s. It's our hope that the Corselet Harness will cause a resurgence of corselet enthusiasm and use. We envision a corselet-wearing army of women and men marching forth in the name of style and reinforced support! Then again...we'd also settle for your bedroom enjoyment of the piece, giving new meaning to the expression, "laid to waist."

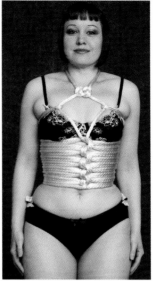 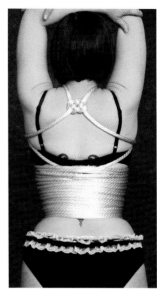

Rope length: 40 to 50 feet (12 – 15m)
Rope diameter: ⅜ to ⁷⁄₁₆ inch (9 – 11mm)

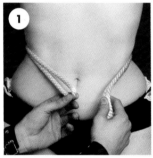

Start by making a bight at the middle of your rope. Hold this bight at the spot on the waist you'd like the corselet to begin.

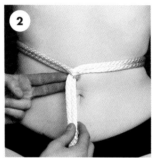

Tuck both working ends through the bight. Then bring the working ends back in the direction they came from, wrapping them all the way around your partner's back...

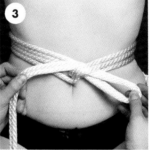

until they reach the bight they created. Once the working ends are back where they started, tuck them both through the bight they created.

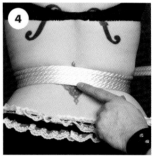

Adjust the tension here to the tightness desired for the piece.

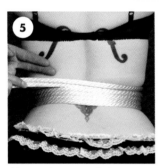

Also make sure all the ropes lined up in the back are parallel to the others.

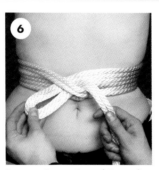

Repeat Steps 2 and 3 until...

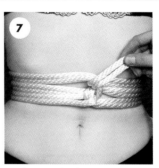

you've worked your way up...

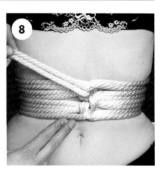

your partner's waist.

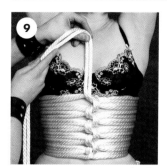

Pause once you've reached the top.

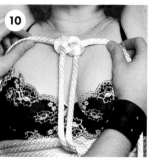

Now draw your working ends up and tie a Double Coin Knot on your partner's chest, lined up between her armpits.

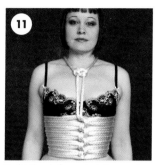

Split the left and right working ends over the neck.

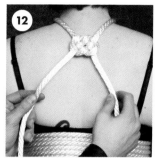

Tie a second Double Coin Knot between the shoulder blades.

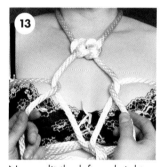

Now split the left and right working ends toward the front of your partner. Tuck them under the vertical ropes beneath the Double Coin Knot. Split the vertical ropes.

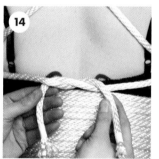

Finally, return the left and right working ends to the back, cross the working ends atop the coils of rope around your partner's waist and...

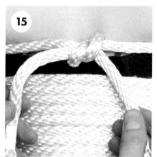

finish the piece by securing the working ends with a Square Knot.

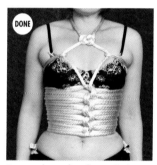

For a clean finish, tuck the Square Knot under the top-most coils of rope in the back.

Pony Harness

Horsing around with your partner is made easy with the help of this stylishly designed chest harness. Using extended and closed Double Coin Knots to create a supportive and comfortable framework of rope, this piece puts power and control into a "trainer's" hands. With a firm tug of the reins, your nay-saying partner will turn giddy for you!

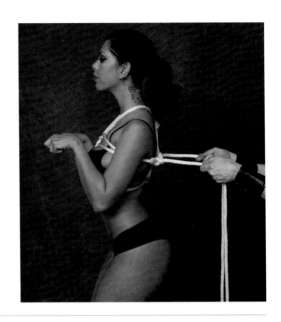

Rope length: 50 feet (15m)
Rope diameter: ³⁄₈ to ⁷⁄₁₆ inch (9 – 11mm)

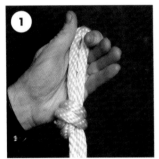

Make a bight in the middle of your rope. Tie a Double Overhand Knot approximately one hand's width from the end of the bight.

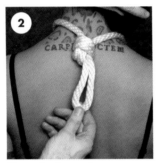

Place the knotted rope around the back of your partner's neck...

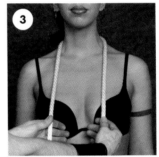

with one rope on each side hanging down from the neck.

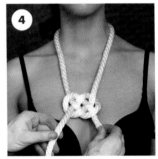

Loosely tie a Double Coin Knot on the upper chest, level with your partner's armpits.

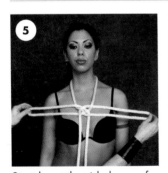

Stretch out the side loops of the Double Coin Knot, about an arm's width wider than the arms, and have your partner hold these bight-like loops in place under the arms.

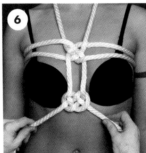

Tie another Double Coin Knot, this time under the breast line.

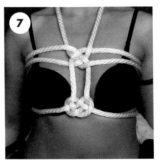

Pass the ropes around to the back on each side of the torso.

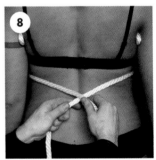

Cross the ropes at the center of the back...

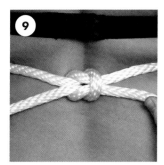

and tie them together with a Square Knot. When tying the Square Knot, be sure to maintain the tightness of both ropes around the torso.

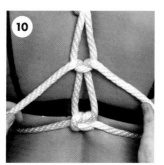

Flip the Square Knot upside down and bring both long ropes through the loop that hangs down from the neck, pulling them from behind toward you.

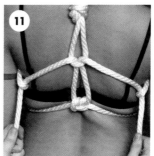

Fish the rope on each side through the bight that's under the armpit. Maintain tension on these ropes.

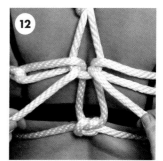

Bring these ropes to the loop again, along and under the previous ropes. Bring them through he loop, from behind toward you.

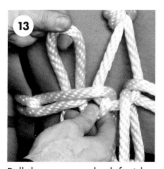

Pull the rope on the left side under and behind the pair of ropes between the loop and the armpit.

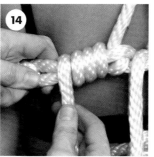

Begin winding the long rope around this pair of ropes, from the loop to the armpit.

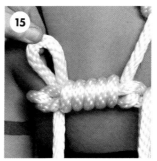

When you reach the bight at the armpit, tie off the winding by lifting a small bight behind and above the winding...

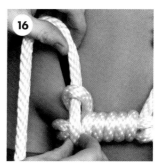

and pulling the end of the rope through this bight.

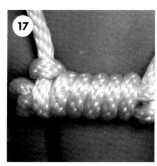

Pull the rope all the way through to collapse the bight onto the rope, securing the piece.

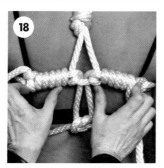

Do the same winding on the right side. Make sure the width of each winding is equal, by measuring or counting the number of winds on each side.

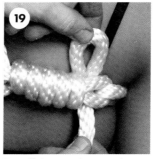

Tie off the winding on the right side, again by lifting a small bight from behind and above...

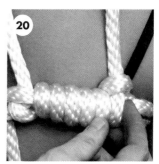

and slipping the long rope through this bight and cinching it tight.

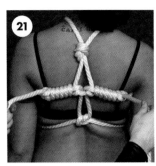 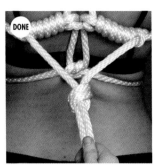 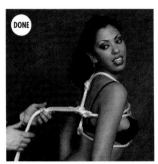 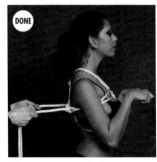

Bring these harness ropes back toward you and begin reining supreme.

You can also tie both ropes together with an Overhand Knot, forming a triangle with equal lengths on each side...

to control your partner singlehandedly.

Now your new little pony can finally start pulling his or her own weight...or yours!

Butterfly Harness

The Butterfly Harness is based on the Long Knot. Left to its own devices, the Long Knot is, well, long. However, when the knot's middle loops are spread wide, it takes on the appearance of the delicate winged creature known collectively as the butterfly. In all truth, the displayed knot could also be said to look like a moth. But the name "Moth Harness" doesn't have the same panache.

Rope length: 30 to 40 feet (9 – 12m)
Rope diameter: ³/₈ to ⁷/₁₆ inch (9 – 11mm)

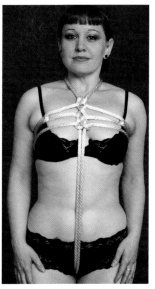
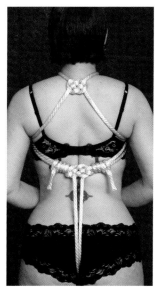

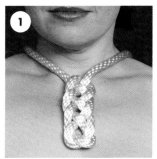

1 Start by tying a Long Knot at the middle of your rope. Drape the left and right working ends of rope over either side of your partner's neck.

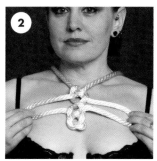

2 Spread the middle loops of the Long Knot out about 3 inches (8cm). Have your partner hold these loops in place.

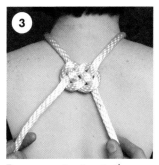

3 Turn your attention to the back of your partner, and tie a Double Coin Knot between the shoulder blades.

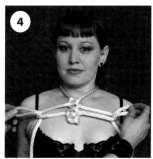

4 Spilt the left and right working ends apart and back toward the front of your partner, tucking each under the left and right "wings" of the Long Knot, respectively.

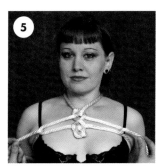

5 Bight the left and right working ends back, wrapping them around the chest.

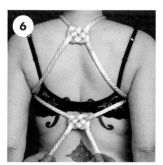

6 When the left and right working ends meet up at the spine, tie a Double Coin Knot.

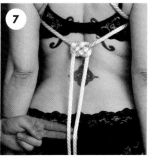

7 Now, drop both working ends down, pulling them up the other side between the legs.

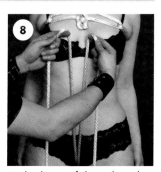

8 At the base of the splayed Long Knot, tuck the left and right working ends under...

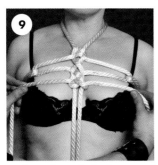

and out through the bottom of the left and right loops. Spilt the working ends apart and bight them toward the back.

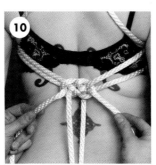

When the left and right working ends return to the spine, tuck each one through the lower loop of the Double Coin Knot.

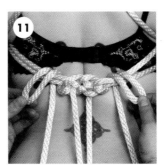

Begin winding one of the working ends around the two horizontal ropes above it.

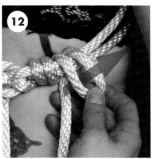

Do this twice. Then tuck a "rabbit ear" (or bight) under the winds, slipping its working end through the back of the loop you created.

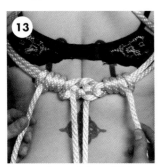

Repeat Steps 11 and 12 on the other side.

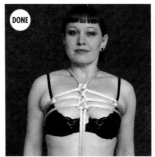

At this point, you can tie off the arms of your partner, or...

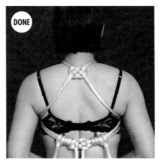

the piece can remain a stand-alone harness.

Lover's Harness

The basis of the Lover's Harness is the True Lover's Knot. Note: although we designed this harness for lovers, you need not be in love, nor have made love, with the person you're tying. That said, you should at least like the person you're tying. If you find yourself disliking the person you're tying, please put your rope down and leave the room.

Rope length: 40 to 50 feet (12 – 15m)
Rope diameter: ³/₈ to ⁷/₁₆ inch (9 – 11mm)

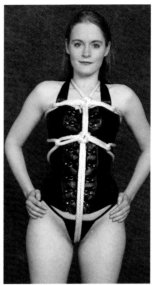
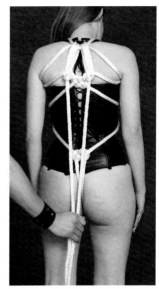

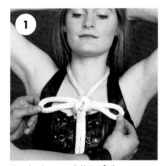

1 With the middle of the rope draped around the back of your partner's neck, tie a True Lover's Knot lined up with your partner's armpits.

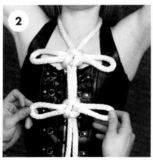

2 About 6 inches (15cm) down from the first True Lover's Knot tie another one.

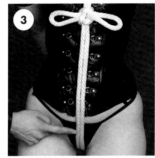

3 Now drop your working ends of rope down and between the legs of your partner.

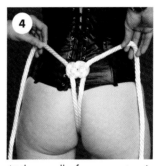

4 At the small of your partner's back tie a Double Coin Knot.

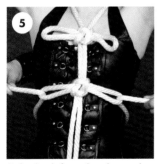

5 Split the left and right working ends toward the front and tuck them under the left and right loops of the lower True Lover's Knot. Bight both ends back again.

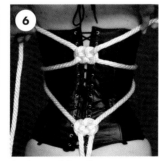

6 At the middle of your partner's back, tie a second Double Coin Knot.

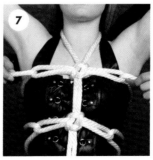

7 Repeat Step 5, only this time, use the top True Lover's Knot.

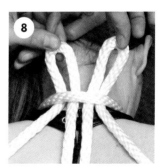

8 Returning your attention to the back of your partner, tuck a pair of "rabbit ears" (or bights) under the rope wrapped around the back of the neck.

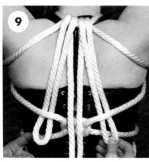

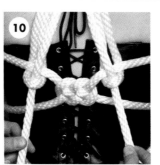

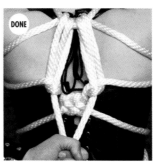

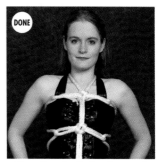

Draw your left and right "rabbit ears" down and under the top of the X at the middle of the back.

Tuck the left and right working ends through the left and right protruding loops, respectively.

Pull the working ends up to cinch the piece in place.

When finished, the front of your lover (or friend, whichever the case may be) should look like this.

Standard Tie-Off

The Standard Tie-Off is for those who can cross their arms behind themselves without discomfort. As the name implies, it's the standard means of restricting vertical (or up and down) movement and lends itself to being incorporated into nearly all of our harnesses. Still, the Standard Tie-Off isn't for everyone, so check out our Limited Flexibility Tie-Off if you face challenges when trying to tie a less limber partner.

Note: This tie-off, as well as the Limited Flexibility option on the next page, can be used in combination with any harness where the working ends dangle down from above.

Rope length: 3 to 5 feet (1 – 1.5m)
Rope diameter: ³/₈ to ⁷/₁₆ inch (9 – 11mm)

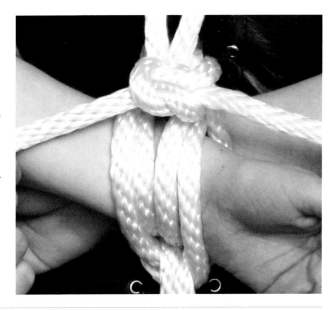

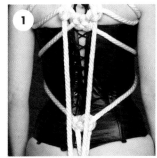

With the chest piece secured, drop the working ends of rope down so that they dangle.

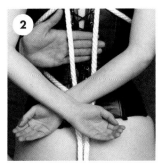

Cross your partner's wrists over the dangling working ends.

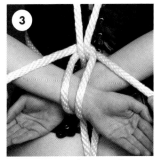

Wrap the working ends around the wrists and up, crossing them behind the vertical ropes between the chest harness and the wrists.

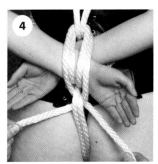

Drop the working ends down over both wrists and cross them behind the rope below.

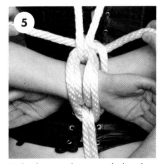

Split the working ends back up, crossing one in front of the back wrist and one behind the front wrist. Cross the ends behind the vertical ropes leading up to the chest.

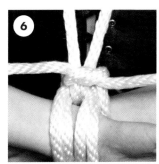

Finish the tie-off with a Split Square Knot.

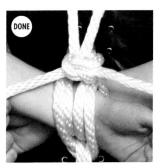

Add an overhand knot for extra security (in case your partner tries anything underhanded).

Limited Flexibility Tie-Off

The Limited Flexibility Tie-Off is for those who cannot cross their arms behind themselves comfortably. The Standard Tie-Off is fine and dandy, but let's face it, not everyone can cross their arms in such a way. Nor should they have to in order to enjoy a fun-filled night of rope play! With respect to this, we present the following option that is equally restrictive but far more comfortable.

Note: This tie-off, as well as the Standard Tie-Off option on the previous page, can be used in combination with any harness where the working ends dangle down from above.

Rope length: 5 to 7 feet (1.5 – 2m)
Rope diameter: ³⁄₈ to ⁷⁄₁₆ inch (9 – 11mm)

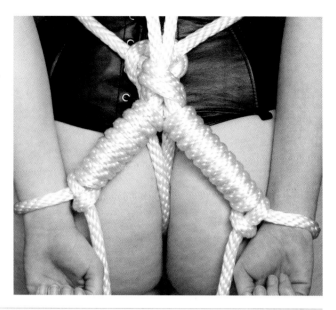

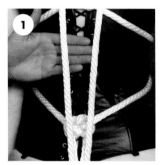

1 With the chest piece secured, drop the working ends of rope down so that they dangle.

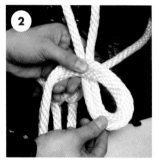

2 Gather the ropes into a pair and rotate them up and over themselves into a counterclockwise circle. Make sure the "leg" of the loop is in front of the *P* shape this creates.

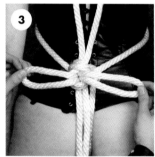

3 Finish this loop off by tying a Double Slipknot.

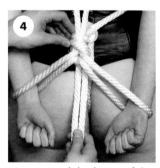

4 Now extend the loops of the Double Slipknot until they reach the position where the wrists are comfortably flexed. Slide the wrists into the loop ends.

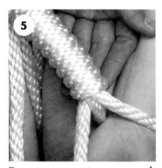

5 Turn your attention to one of the loops and start coiling your corresponding working end of the rope around it until it is one wind from the wrist.

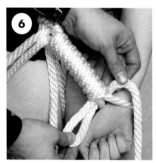

6 Create a "rabbit ear" (or bight) above the wrist.

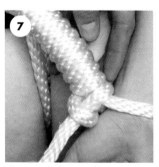

7 Then tuck the working end into the loop created.

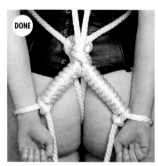

DONE Repeat Steps 5 through 7 on the other side and you're done!

Advanced Harnesses

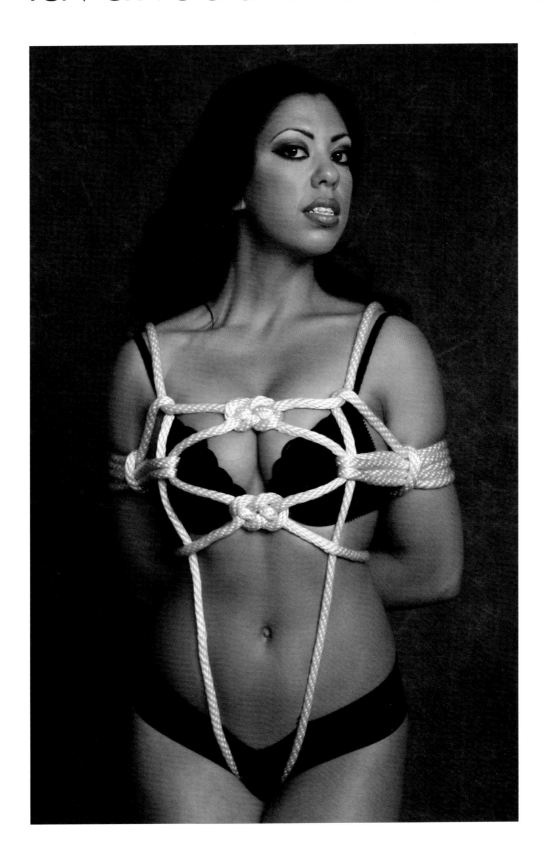

Hip Harness

Want to keep your partner's ass up while maintaining her exposed and sexually available? Well, here we show how you do it! Effectively a climbing harness that was modified to maintain sexual accessibility, this tie is one of our most popular. Not only does it easily adjust to the size of the person being tied, it's comfortable, stable and allows for hours of raucous play—or even more uplifting activities.

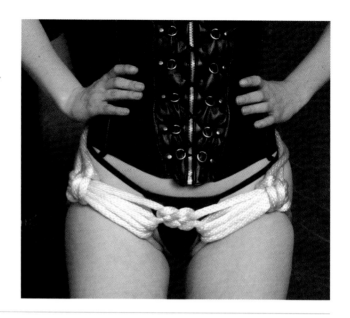

Rope length: 40 to 60 feet (12 – 18m)
Rope diameter: 3/8 to 7/16 inch (9 – 11mm)

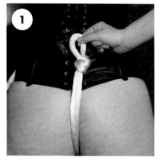

Start by measuring a fistance (a fist distance) down from the bight of the middle of the rope. At the base of the fistance, tie a Double Overhand Knot.

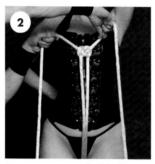

As your partner holds the Overhand Knot at the base of the spine, bring the two working ends up between the legs to the middle of the chest. Tie a Double Coin Knot.

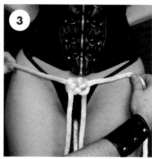

Drop the Double Coin Knot down to your partner's belly. Then split the left and right working ends of the rope, taking one over each hip.

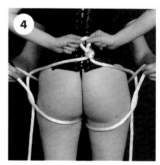

Tuck the left and right working ends UNDER the ropes that lead down from the Double Overhand Knot.

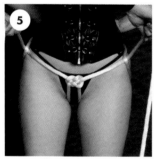

Bight the working ends toward the front of your partner.

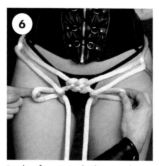

In the front, tuck the working ends OVER the parallel ropes below the Double Coin Knot and bight them back again.

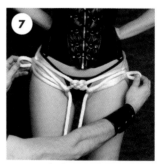

Now tuck the working ends UNDER the ropes on the side of the hips...

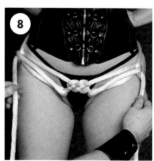

and bight them back to the front again.

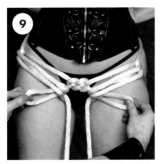

Continue winding back and forth, OVER the ropes below the Double Coin Knot...

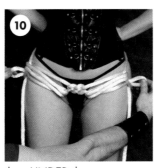

then UNDER the ropes alongside the hips...

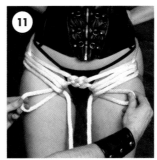

and OVER the ropes below the Double Coin Knot again.

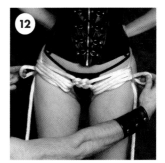

Tuck the working ends UNDER a fourth time. The winds of rope should measure equally on each side. Adjust them if needed, but don't cinch the harness too tightly.

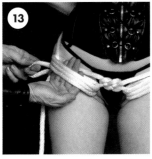

If you've woven the working ends correctly (under the back and over the front), you should be able to run your hand between winds without hitting a crossed rope.

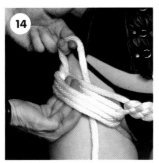

If you feel crossed ropes, undo the winds and adjust your harness before moving on. To secure the winding in place, tuck the working end under all the winds...

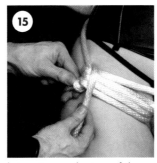

bring it over the top of those winds...

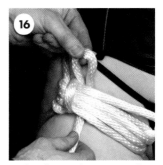

and pull it under again. This second time, leave a "rabbit ear" (or bight) sticking out from the top.

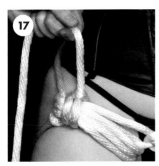

Push the working end through the "rabbit ear" and pull it tight.

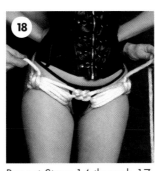

Repeat Steps 14 through 17 on the other hip.

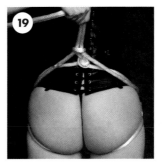

Now bring both working ends back toward the loop you created when you tied the Double Overhand Knot. Pull the ropes completely through the loop as shown.

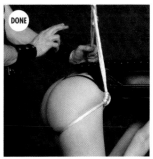

Now just tie your ropes to a secure point above your partner's head. When bending over, your partner's hips stay in the perfect position for spanking or (ahem) more!

Side Arm Harness

This tie was inspired by the engineering of a corset. Simple yet effective, the corset maintains restriction in a way that begs to be emulated for the purpose of functional bondage. The Side Arm Harness provides that restriction of the body and arms while still allowing use of your partner's forearms and hands.

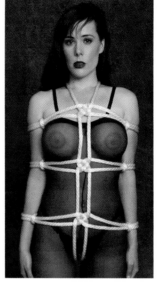
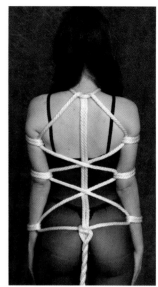

Rope length: 40 to 60 feet (12 – 18m)
Rope diameter: 3/8 to 7/16 inch (9 – 11mm)

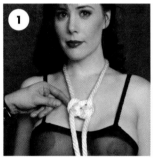

Start by tying a Double Coin Knot in the middle of your partner's chest.

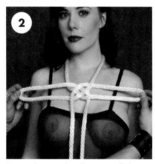

Stretch out the loops of the Double Coin Knot...

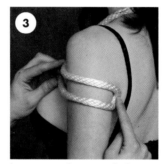

long enough to reach the shoulder blades of the person you're tying.

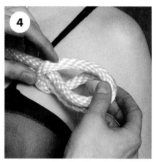

Create a bight that folds forward onto itself.

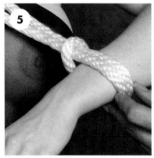

Have your partner slip a wrist through the loop that you created.

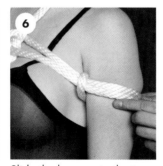

Slide the loop up to the top of your partner's arm. This loop, and all the ones to follow, should maintain a two-finger space between the rope and the skin.

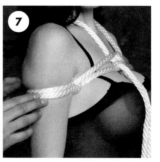

Repeat Steps 4 through 6 on the other arm.

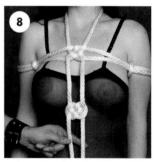

Below the chest line, tie a second Double Coin Knot.

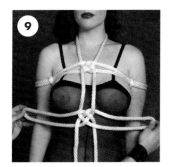

Again, stretch out the loops of the Double Coin Knot...

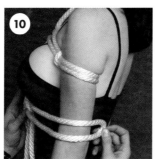

long enough to line up with the shoulder blades of the person you're tying.

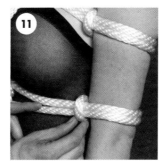

Create a loop and slide it into place, this time just above the elbow.

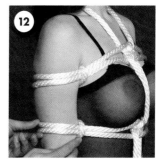

Repeat Steps 9 through 11 on the other arm.

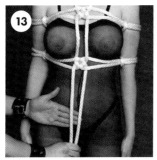

At this point your piece should look like this.

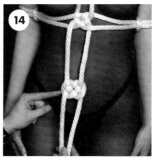

Atop the belly button of your partner, tie a third Double Coin Knot.

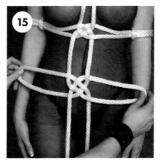

Once again, stretch the loops out long, only this time make sure their ends reach the left and right hips of your partner.

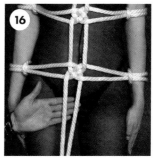

Create loops, just as before, and slide your partner's wrists into place.

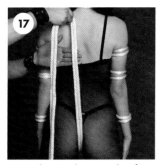

Drop the working ends of rope down between the legs and up the back of your partner.

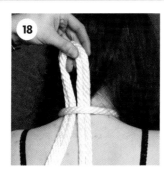

Tuck the working ends underneath the rope around your partner's neck.

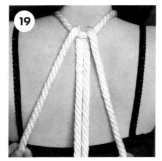

Split the working ends apart.

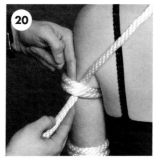

Tuck each working end behind the left...

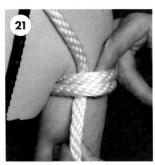

and right upper arm wrap, respectively.

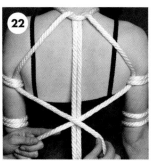

After crossing the ropes across your partner's back...

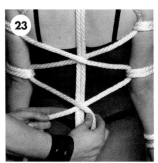

repeat Steps 20 and 21 for the elbow wraps...

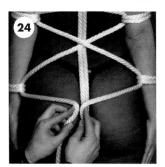

and the forearm wraps.

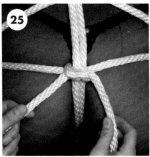

Finish the piece off with a Split Square Knot.

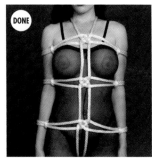

Standing at attention...

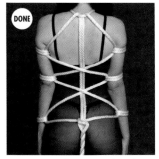

was never this easy (or disarmingly beautiful)!

Modified Pearls

One step beyond our Japanese Pearl Harness, the Modified Pearls restricts the arms from flexing forward through the use of a stretched diamond rig across the back. The addition of this rig further impedes escape, but doesn't change the fundamental structure of the tie. The breasts will still be pinched between the ropes stretched across the chest and maintain their "string of pearls" appearance.

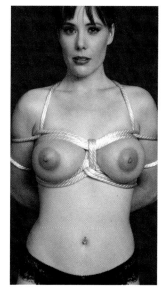
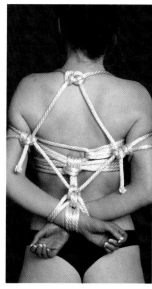

Rope length: 40 to 60 feet (12 – 18m)
Rope diameter: ⅜ to ⁷⁄₁₆ inch (9 – 11mm)

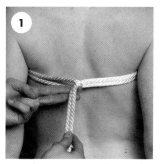

1 Start by wrapping the working ends around the top of your partner's chest (above the breasts) and tucking them through a bight positioned along the spine.

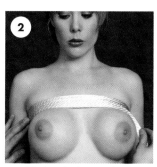

2 Double back the working ends, wrapping them around the chest, just below the first wrap. Adjust the tension to make the wraps firm, but not uncomfortably tight.

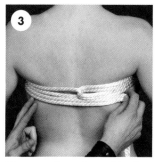

3 Once you've returned to the line of the spine, wrap the working ends around the chest a third time...

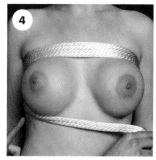

4 only this rotation should wrap below the breasts instead of above them.

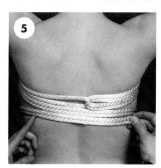

5 Again, wrap the working ends around. Only this time...

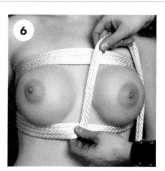

6 pause at the middle of the lowest row of ropes in the front. Make a backward L shape.

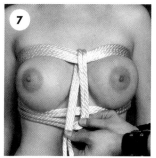

7 Draw the working ends up and over the top rows...

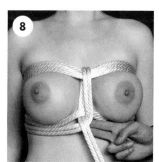

8 and underneath the lowest row of ropes. Then, pull the working ends out the front through the corner of the L.

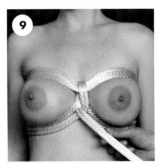

9

At this point, pulling the working ends firmly will squeeze the breasts together like a string of pearls. Continue wrapping around toward the back.

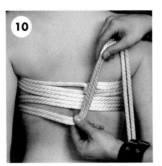

10

Along the spine, make another backward L, tucking the working ends...

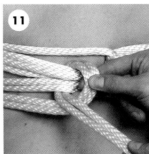

11

through the original bight, behind the top rows of rope and forward through the corner of the L.

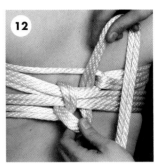

12

Curl the working ends forward, around the hook of the L, up behind the all the rows and out through the original bight.

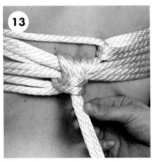

13

Bring the working ends down and tuck them through the loop created by the curl made at the base of the wraps.

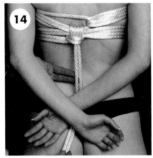

14

The chest piece now secured, cross your partner's wrists over the dangling working ends of rope.

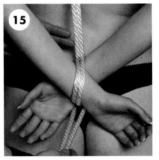

15

Wrap the working ends around the wrists and then up...

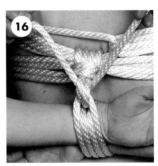

16

crossing them behind the vertical ropes between the chest harness and the wrists.

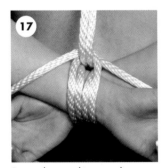

17

Drop the working ends down, crossing one end behind the wrist in the back and the other behind the wrist in the front.

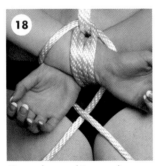

18

Cross the working ends at the bottom of the wrists...

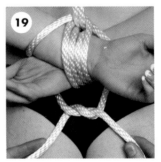

19

and tie an Overhand Knot.

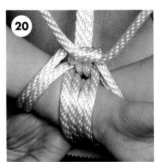

20

Bring the working ends back up and tie a Split Square Knot around the vertical ropes between the chest harness and the wrists.

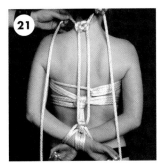

21 Draw the working ends of the rope up and over the back of the chest harness. Make a Double Coin Knot just below the neckline.

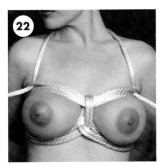

22 Split the working ends apart over your partner's shoulders, tucking the left and right working ends under the left and right top row of rope, respectively.

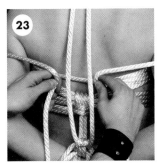

23 After splitting the working ends apart and returning them to the back, tuck the left and right working ends...

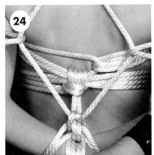

24 under the left and right parallel ropes between the neck and the wrists. Pull the parallel ropes apart.

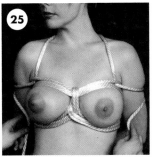

25 Wrap the left and right working ends around...

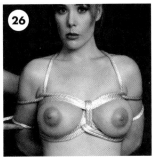

26 the left and right upper arms. Make sure to leave a two-finger space between the wound rope and the upper arms.

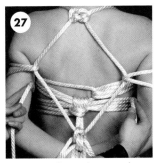

27 Wrap each working end...

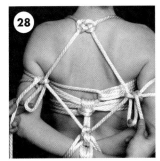

28 once around the horizontal rope above each, respectively. Then tuck a "rabbit ear" (or bight) out from the bottom of the horizontal rope.

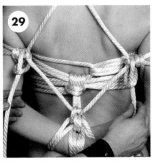

29 Slip each working end into its respective "rabbit ear" and...

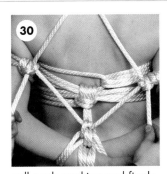

30 pull each working end firmly.

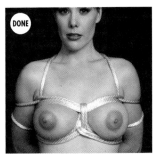

DONE The finished piece looks like this from the front...

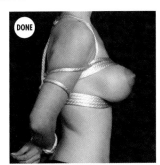

DONE and like this from the side.

Chest Plate Harness

This is a sturdy harness with an elegant front and a deceptively complex back. The front of the piece is supported by the Prosperity Knot, a knot that in addition to its beauty also distributes weight extremely well. The back of the piece is the result of a dynamic weave that allows spring when struggled against. As far as esthetic, functional ties go, this is one of our favorites!

Rope length: 40 to 50 feet (12 – 15m)
Rope diameter: ³/₈ to ⁷/₁₆ inch (9 – 11mm)

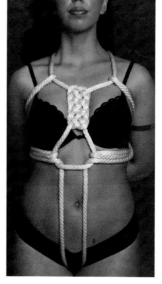
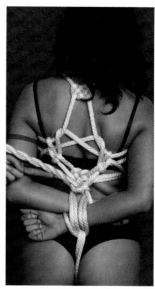

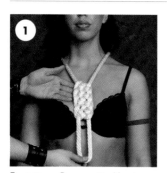

1 First tie a Prosperity Knot one fistance down from the middle of your rope. Drape the left and right working ends over the left and right shoulder of your partner, respectively.

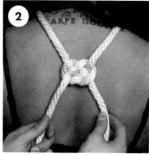

2 Tie a Double Coin Knot between your partner's shoulders.

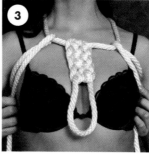

3 Split the left and right working ends toward the front. Tuck them under the left and right side of the loop ABOVE the Prosperity Knot and bight the working ends back.

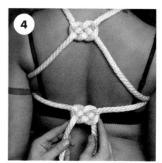

4 Bring the working ends together along the spine and tie a second Double Coin Knot. Make the knot firm but not too tight. Split the left and right ends back toward the front.

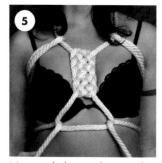

5 Now tuck the working ends underneath the left and right side of the loop BELOW the Prosperity Knot and bight them back again.

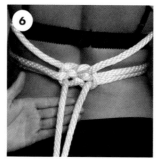

6 Tuck the left and right working ends through the left and right loops of the Double Coin Knot. Then, drop the working ends down...

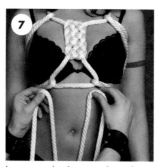

7 between the legs and up the front, pausing at the base of the loop below the Prosperity Knot. Make sure your working ends don't cross and remain parallel to one another.

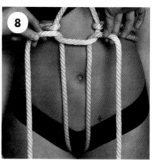

8 Tuck the left and right working ends under the loop below the Prosperity Knot, splitting the working ends apart and...

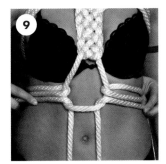

toward the back.

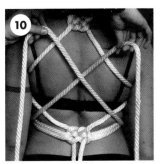

Cross the working ends across your partner's back...

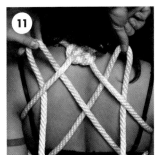

then tuck a "rabbit ear" (or bight) of the left and right working end under the ropes that branch off the bottom of the first Double Coin Knot.

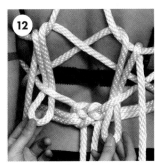

Now drop the left and right "rabbit ears" down and tuck them beneath the ropes branching off the top of the second Double Coin Knot.

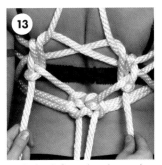

Tuck the left and right working ends through their respective loops and pull the piece together firmly.

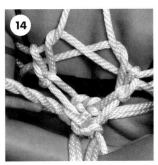

At this point, you can perform the Standard Tie-Off (shown) or the Limited Flexibility Tie-Off.

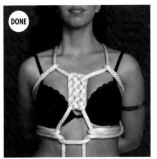

Although your Chest Plate Harness won't protect your partner during a medieval joust...

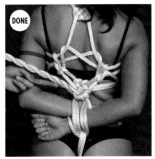

it's great for a night of medieval-themed passion and play!

Star Back Harness

The perfect harness for "squirmy" bottoms who claim they can get out of anything, the Star Back is as effective as it is beautiful. Utilizing vertical and horizontal suppression of the upper arms and wrists in order to maintain its control, the tie, once finished, results in an appealing front design and the appearance of a "star" on the back of the person tied.

Rope length: 40 to 50 feet (12 – 15m)
Rope diameter: 3/8 to 7/16 inch (9 – 11mm)

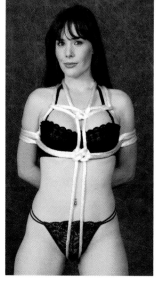
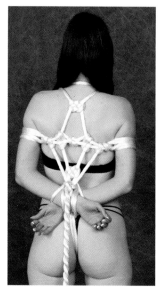

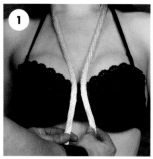

Begin the piece by draping the middle of the rope over the back of your partner's neck.

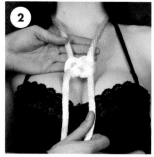

Tie a Double Coin Knot in the middle of your partner's chest.

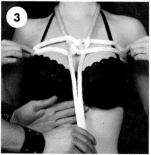

Pull the left and right loops of the Double Coin Knot apart. Have your partner hold the loops in place in front of the armpits.

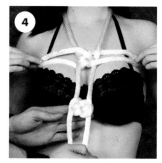

About two inches (5cm) down from the first Double Coin Knot, tie a second one.

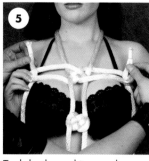

Tuck both working ends up through the loops of the first Double Coin Knot, and drape them over your partner's shoulders.

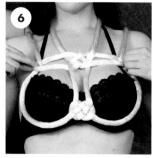

There should now be two large loops circling your partner's chest.

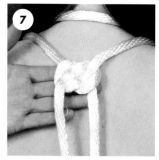

Turn your attention to your partner's back. Tie a Double Coin Knot between the shoulder blades.

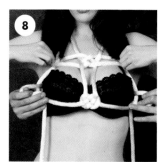

Then, bring the working ends back toward the front of your partner and tuck them underneath the left and right loops circling her chest.

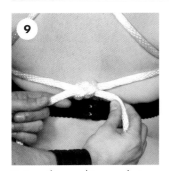

Return the working ends to the back and tie a taut Square Knot.

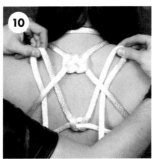

Now tuck "rabbit ears" (or bights) under the ropes branching off the bottom of the Double Coin Knot.

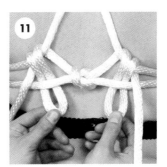

Pull the two "rabbit ears" down and tuck them underneath the ropes branching off the bottom of the Square Knot.

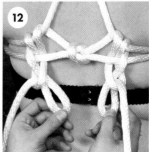

Tuck the left and right working ends through the left and right "rabbit ears" and...

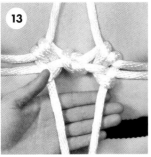

cinch them down firmly.

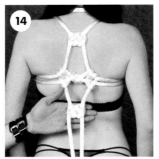

About two inches (5cm) below the cinched rope, tie another Double Coin Knot.

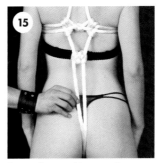

Drop the working ends down between the legs...

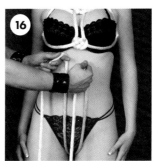

and bring them up to the lower Double Coin Knot on the chest. Make sure the working ends remain parallel to each other.

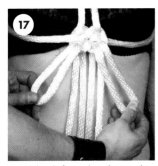

Tuck the left and right working ends through the left and right bottom loops of the Double Coin Knot, respectively.

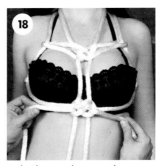

Split the working ends apart, toward the back.

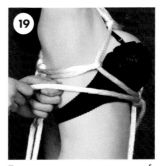

Turn your attention to one of the working ends. Bring it under the arm of your partner, who should drop the arm onto the rope once you bring it around.

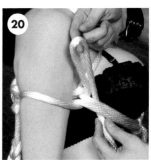

Then bring the working end over the upper arm, underneath and out the top of the horizontal ropes in the front.

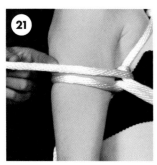

Bring the working end back again, over the upper arm. Note: all these winds should maintain a two-finger space between the rope and the skin.

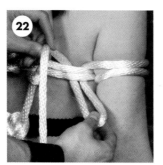

This time, tuck the working end over the top and out the bottom of the horizontal ropes in the back.

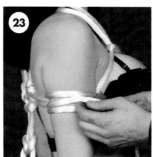

Bring the working end back toward the front, splitting it between the two horizontal ropes that wind around the arm.

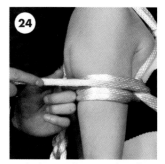

Tuck the working end underneath and out the top of the horizontal ropes in the front.

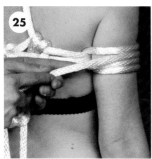

Bring the working end back one more time, making sure to press it between the first and the second rope winds around the arm when you do.

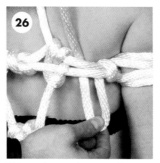

Wrap the working end around the horizontal ropes in the back, tucking a "rabbit ear" (or bight) under the ropes adjacent to the first vertical wind.

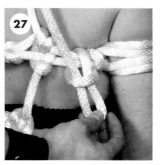

Now tuck the working end through the "rabbit ear."

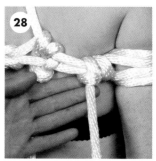

Pull the working end firmly to lock everything in place.

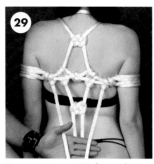

Repeat Steps 19 through 28 on the other side. Remember to maintain a two-finger space between all the winds of the rope and the skin.

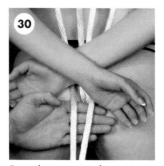

From here onward, you can either tie the Limited Flexibility Tie-Off, or...

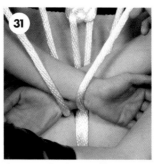

the Standard Tie-Off...

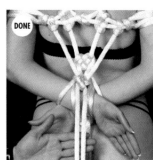

as shown here.

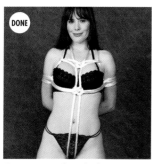

Once completed, the tie should look like this in the front...

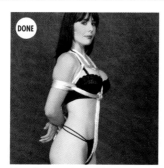

like this on the right...

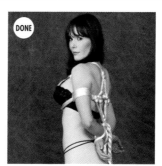

like this on the left...

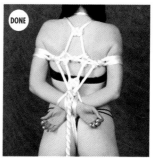

and like this in the back. If you did it right, you can make a wish upon your lucky star!

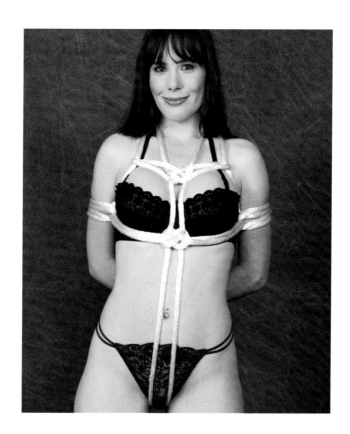

Stacker Harness

This is an example of a modified Japanese "*Hon Kikkou*" tie (*Kikkou* is the Japanese word for tortoise). Tied with one continuous strip of rope, the piece holds its decorative look and maintains its effectiveness during struggle. We gave our version of the *Hon Kikkou* the name "Stacker" on account of the stacked Double Coin Knots that appear on the back of the finished piece. It works especially well if your partner also happens to be nicely stacked.

Rope length: 40 to 50 feet (12 – 15m)
Rope diameter: ³⁄₈ to ⁷⁄₁₆ inch (9 – 11mm)

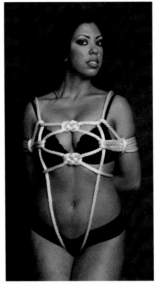
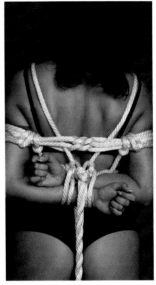

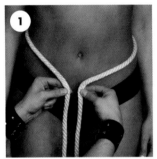

1 Start with the middle of the rope wrapped around the back of your partner's waist. Pinch the working ends of the rope together at your partner's belly and...

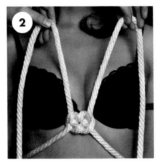

2 tie a Double Coin Knot so that it sits just below the chest line.

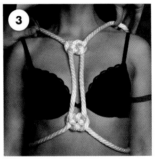

3 Tie a second Double Coin Knot above the chest line.

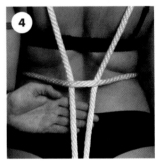

4 Bring the working ends over the shoulders, on either side of the neck, and under the rope wrapped around the waist.

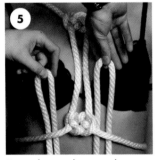

5 Drop the working ends down between the legs and up underneath the ropes stemming from the lower Double Coin Knot.

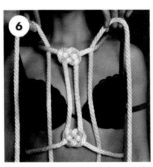

6 Continue up and underneath the ropes stemming from the upper Double Coin Knot.

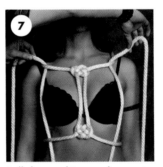

7 Pull the working ends apart toward the outside of your partner's chest.

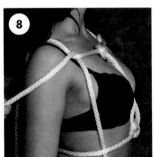

8 Now bring the working ends over the upper arms, around and...

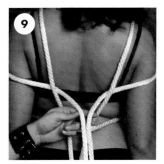

9

underneath the vertical ropes along the back.

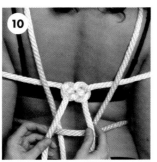

10

Tie a Double Coin Knot between the shoulder blades.

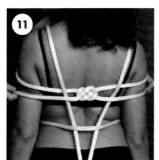

11

Bring the working ends back toward the front of your partner.

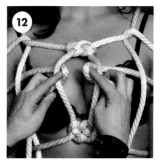

12

Tuck each working end underneath the front vertical ropes and underneath the loop between the upper and lower Double Coin Knots.

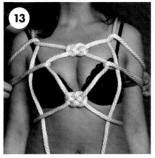

13

Pull the working ends back over the upper arms, around and...

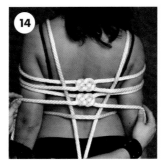

14

underneath the back vertical ropes. Tie a Double Coin Knot below the one above.

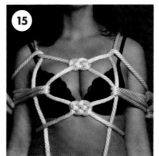

15

Bring the working ends back to the front. Tuck each working end under the front vertical ropes and underneath the loop between the Double Coin Knots.

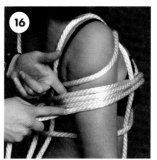

16

Bring one of the working ends toward your partner's back. Pass it over the upper arm. All winds should maintain a two-finger space between the rope and the skin.

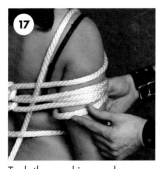

17

Tuck the working end between the body and the upper arm.

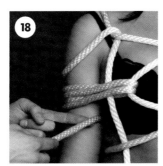

18

The working end should emerge below the front horizontal wraps.

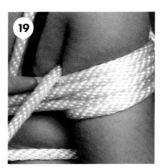

19

Curl the working end up and over the horizontal wraps, then over the top of the back horizontal wraps...

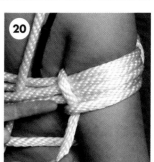

20

and down through the back of the rope that passed between the body and the upper arm.

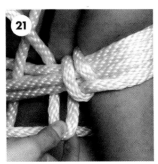

21 Wrap the working end up and around the back horizontal ropes, leaving a "rabbit ear" (or bight) sticking out from the bottom of your wrap.

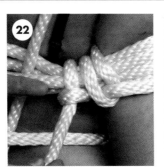

22 Tuck the working end through the "rabbit ear" and lock the loop in place.

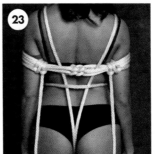

23 Repeat Steps 16 though 22 on the other side. Remember: maintain a two-finger space between all the winds of rope and the skin.

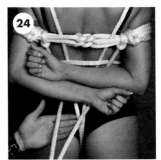

24 Now have your partner place both arms behind the back, laying them over the working ends of the rope and gripping her forearms as best she can (if she can).

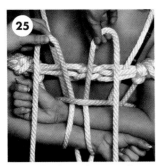

25 Wrap both working ends up and underneath the rope wrapped around the waist.

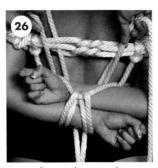

26 Bring the working ends down, back around the forearms.

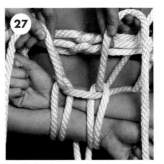

27 Tuck the left and right working ends though the left and right loops at the wrists, respectively.

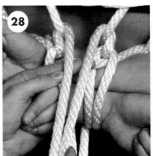

28 Pull the working ends up and wrap them around the back of the left and right vertical ropes along the back.

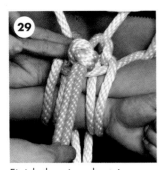

29 Finish the piece by tying a Double Overhand Knot. Congratulations—you just finished the toughest tie in the book!

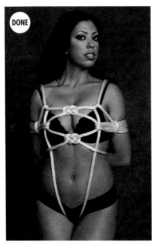

Front view!

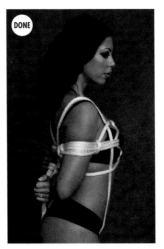

Side view!

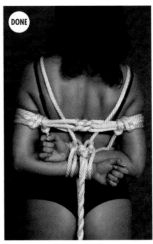

Back view!

Glossary

bend

Strictly speaking, a bend is any knot that joins two ropes together. Therefore, we should note that the Sliding Sheet Bend is not technically a bend, but gets its name from its *resemblance* to the Sheet Bend. Rather than being academic purists, we let its name slide.

bight

A *U*-shaped semicircle of rope where the rope does not cross itself. It can be used to assist in the tying of a knot when rope length would make using the actual end of the rope impractical or awkward.

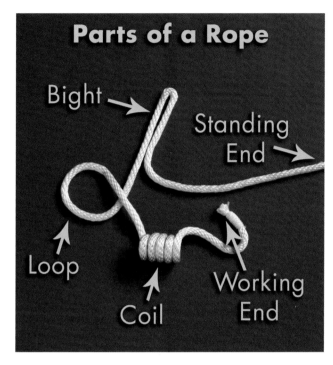

Parts of a Rope

Bight →

Standing End →

Loop

Coil

Working End

coil

To wind into continuous, regularly spaced spirals or rings, one beside the other. Also a key part of the name from several bands JD and Dan enjoy (Coil, Icon of Coil, Lacuna Coil, This Mortal Coil, *et al*).

corselet

An undergarment that combines a girdle and a bra. Although still in use, corselets were more popular from the mid-1910s through the 1950s.

fistance

The fusion of the words "fist" and "distance," a fistance is an approximate unit of measurement represented by the distance between your thumb-knuckle and your pinky-knuckle when making a fist.

flying your flag

A slang term that means to show what kink you have in a public setting, usually by a particular style of dress, or through the use of colored bandanas. "Flying one's flag" is a way to meet up with like-minded people.

Hana Musubi

In Japanese the word "Hana" means flower and the word "Musubi" means to connect, end or bind together. Together the words Hana Musubi roughly translate to "flower tying" or when referring to rope work the appearance of a Flower Knot.

Hojojutsu

The technique used in feudal Japan to restrain prisoners with rope. Hojojutsu is usually not taught on its own but instead as part of a more expanded martial arts curriculum. However, due to the relatively recent upwelling of interest in sensual rope bondage, there are now educators (primarily in the United States) who have studied and now teach this ancient technique on its own.

Hon Kikkou

A Japanese term that refers to a weaving design in fabric that looks like a tortoise shell. In the context of rope bondage it describes a tortoise shell shaped pattern of rope used to beautify the person being tied while restraining the arms against the torso.

loop

A circle of rope in which the rope crosses itself.

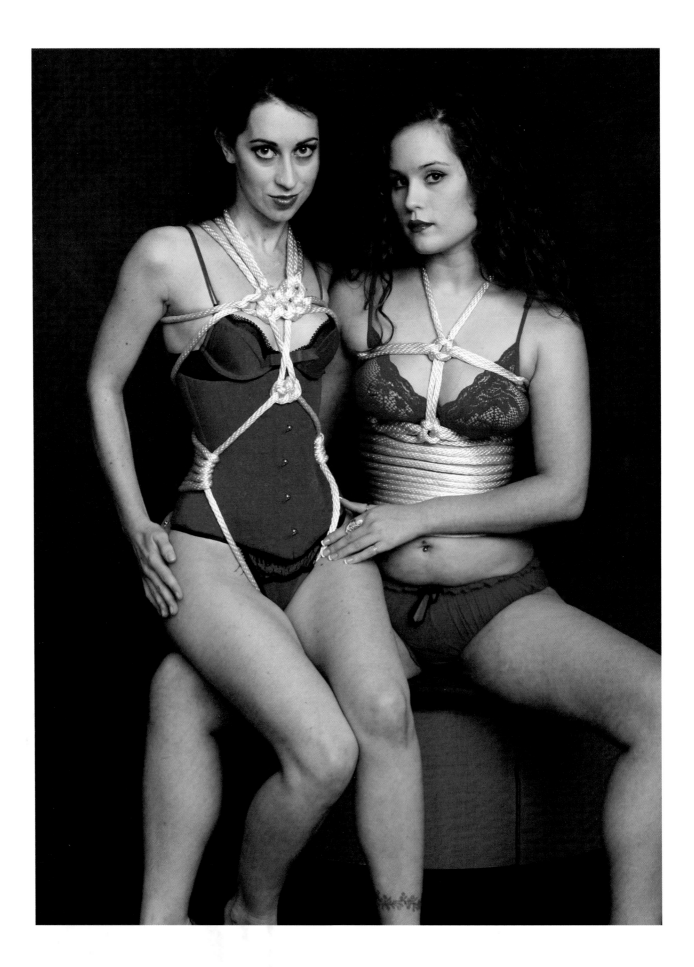

obi

The Japanese word that refers to several different types of sashes worn with traditional Japanese clothing. In the United States this is more popularly known as the belt worn in judo, aikido and karate. Also the name that only Obi Wan Kenobi's parents or lovers could get away with calling him without risk of sudden death by light saber.

pigeon toe

Also called "in-toeing," it is an orientation of the hips and knees that allows the toes to point inward. Such a position can be used to inhibit sexual accessibility.

rabbit ears

The name we give for a bight that sticks out the top or bottom of a length of rope.

rigger

Traditionally the name given to a shipyard worker who fits or dismantles the standing and running lines of ships. However, in more recent years, the term has been assimilated into the sensual rope bondage community to identify any person who formalizes his or her enjoyment of tying people with rope.

rolling rope

The overlapping of one rope across another rope when wound around a body part or object.

Shibari

Literally meaning "to tie," it is a Japanese style of sexual rope restraint. Shibari differs from Western bondage in that, instead of just immobilizing or restraining the bottom, it also gives the bottom pleasure from being under pressure and strain from the ropes squeezing against his or her breasts or genitals. Ironically, the term was popularized in the West (during the 1990s) to describe the Japanese style of restraint.

squirmy bottoms

A term used to described persons who, when tied in rope, get enjoyment from struggling in or resisting their bindings.

standing end

A term used to denote the end of the rope that does not have the knot in it, or is not involved in making the knot.

stupa

A mound-like structure that contains Buddhist relics, typically, the remains of a Buddha or saint. Once places of worship, it is believed that stupas evolved into pagodas, as Buddhism spread from India into other Asian countries.

tie

A single rope bondage technique or application, or a piece that is tied.

two-finger rule

An approximate gauge of space between a tied rope and the body part it encircles. Tying the bondage in a way that maintains enough space to fit one or two fingers between the rope and skin allows consistent blood circulation to flow through the bound area.

weave/weaving

The process of a rope passing alternately over and under each other rope it crosses.

wind/winding

Coiling the rope (in parallel layers) around a body part, object or another rope.

working end

A term used to denote the end of the rope that is used to make the knot or the piece being tied—can also be called the "running end" or "live end."

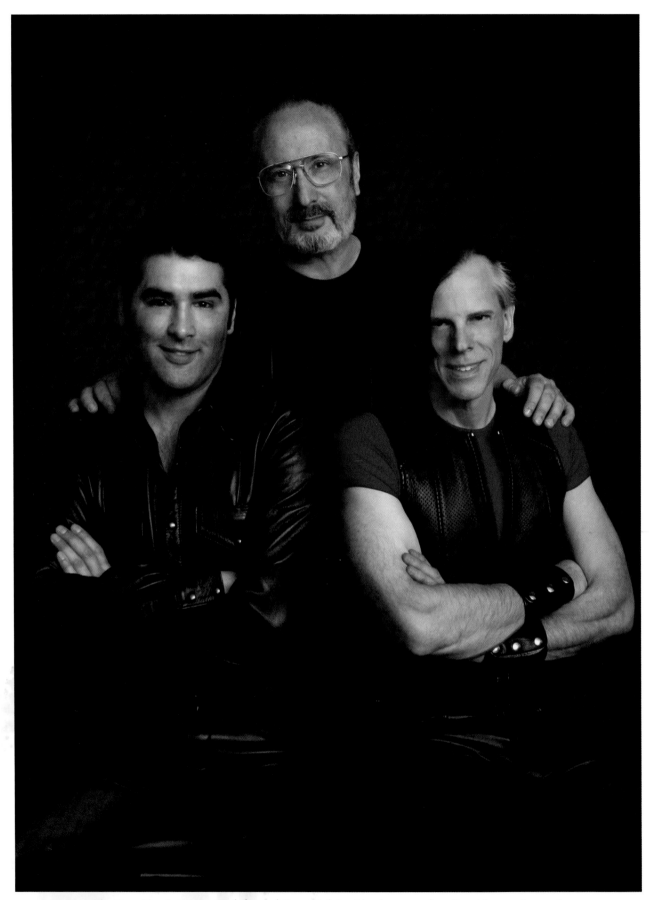

The Two Knotty Boys, JD (left) and Dan (right) with photographer Ken Marcus (center).

About the Authors

The Two Knotty Boys, JD and Dan, combine more than three decades of rope bondage experience, including tying models for world-renowned fetish photographers. Rope bondage blossomed naturally from JD's former work as an industrial rigger and Dan's hobby as a climbing instructor.

Meeting in 1999, as both tied applicants for a bondage-modeling contest, JD and Dan noticed their similarity of bondage styles and philosophy—and they soon joined forces as the Two Knotty Boys. Ever since, they've been performing live shows, rigging photo shoots and teaching bondage to packed workshops worldwide. JD's scientific background and extensive knowledge of human physiology and Dan's mountaineering experience and years of performing stand-up comedy add to their uniquely informative and enjoyable teaching style.

With light-hearted humor and the educational precision of experienced instructors and lifestyle Doms, their impact on the rope bondage scene expanded worldwide with their first best-selling guidebook, *Two Knotty Boys Showing You the Ropes*. Creators of nearly one hundred free video tutorials, JD and Dan are innovative educators and contributors—consistently pushing the boundaries of what can be accomplished with rope.

Photographer Ken Marcus has more than a painstaking eye for detail. He embodies the creativity of an artist with the discipline of a craftsman. He spent thirteen years studying with Ansel Adams, arguably America's photographer laureate. Born in 1946, he studied music and art. As early as age fifteen, while still in secondary school, Ken began taking university-level photography night classes at the Art Center College of Design in Los Angeles.

From black-and-white landscapes, Ken moved to the fast-paced world of glamor and erotic photography, becoming *Penthouse* magazine's first American photographer in 1972. He joined *Playboy* in 1974 as their West Coast Contributing Photographer, shooting centerfolds, editorials and calendars for eleven years—twice receiving their prestigious "Photographer of the Year Award." After leaving *Playboy*, Ken returned to shooting for *Penthouse* and also spent ten years as the cover photographer for *Muscle & Fitness* magazine, plus producing expensive glamor calendars for corporate clients.

Now "officially retired" from the commercial world of photography, Ken immerses himself exclusively in producing images for his website, www.KenMarcus.com. His idea of "retirement" involves shooting erotica two to three days a week.